Praise for The Elep

"What a real gem of a book that li ____ dark corners in the life of many children who struggle to learn — and this will definitely help their parents, teachers and carers to better support these kids and empower them to succeed.

I have first-hand experience of many things she describes...and once there is greater understanding of the challenges these beautiful children face, it is so much easier to feel compassion, empathy and patience rather than frustration! As a School Trustee (the new name for School Governors), I would also recommend this book to teaching staff, simply because the strategies, tools and techniques included are so valuable. Any quick wins that support teachers to empower their students are worth adopting in an educational setting."

Karen Falconer, CEO of the Association for NLP, mum and School Trustee.

"If you are reading this book then you are someone who wants to make a difference. The pages of this book could well hold your very own 'light bulb moment' in how you think about learning and about learning differences. For me, teaching children how to best utilise their mental imagery made so much sense that I couldn't wait to try it out. I am on a journey, keen to learn more and apply [my new knowledge] to all different areas of learning. As an ex-head teacher I am appealing to all forward-thinking school leaders to read this book and lead the way in changing the educational pedagogy so that children labelled with so-called learning 'difficulties' do not need to be subjected to year on year 'interventions' and be made to feel in some way inferior to their peers."

Sally Pattrick: ex-head teacher and SENCo.

"Big challenges are looming in the world. We don't need more frustrated, angry, resigned, or hopeless people. The loss to society of so many talented people who could be contributing to themselves and others is enormous. The loss of the contributions that could have been made by creative people who think differently is impossible to calculate. We need all the neurodivergent students, who think differently, to resolve the challenges of today.

It is time to stop complaining about the problems of education and time to introduce these proven concepts and methods into more and more schools. Do yourself the favour of reading this book, and of giving it to people who need it."

Art Giser, Creator of Energetic NLP.

In this 'upside-down' world, Olive has revealed the scandal of thousands of talented children confined to a world of learning difficulties because they learn differently and do not have access to the simple life altering skill of mental imagery. Her ground-breaking book is the start of an educational revolution.

Dr. Richard De Souza, General Practitioner and Mental Coach.

The Elephants in the Classroom: Uncovering Every Student's Natural Power of Mental Imagery to Enhance Learning

By OLIVE HICKMOTT

www.empoweringlearning.co.uk

Published by
MX Publishing
A New Perspectives Book

**For more information about the book take a look at:
www.tiahl.org and the author's associated practice
www.empoweringlearning.co.uk**

ISBN Paperback 978-1-78705-460-8,
ISBN ePub 978-1-78705-461-5, ISBN PDF 978-1-78705-462-2

First published in 2019
© Copyright 2019
Olive Hickmott

Although every effort has been made to ensure the accuracy of the information contained in this guide as of the date of publication, nothing herein should be construed as giving specific treatment advice. In addition, the application of the techniques to specific circumstances can present complex issues that are beyond the scope of this guide. This publication is intended to provide general information pertaining to developing these skills.

Published in the UK by MX Publishing, 335, Princess Park Manor, Royal Drive, London, N11 3GX (www.mxpublishing.co.uk)

Dedication

I want to dedicate this book to all those bright, creative children and adults who think there is something wrong with them because they don't learn in the way others do. "I should like to change your perspectives; you are exceptional people; creative, imaginative, talented.....with valuable neurodivergent skills and strengths. You are people who can make major changes to the world."

It is my ardent hope this book will alter your view of learning differences and thus allow hundreds of thousands of students to realise their full potential and become life-long learners.

Acknowledgements

There are many people I wish to thank for their help, inspiration, and influence in writing this book:

Among them are Dr Art Giser, creator of Energetic NLP, (www.energeticNLP.com); Ian McDermott; Robert Dilts; Tim Hallbom; Suzi Smith, Robert Fletcher and Peter King for their invaluable training programmes.

Caroline Chapple, www.chapplecoaching.com, for her many fabulous illustrations; she has the great skill to be able to bring my ideas to life on the page and inspired me to add my personal contributions as well.

All those colleagues who have given me feedback on the book, especially the two master trainers, Sara Haboubi and Paula Montie, who have been vital in the development of Empowering Learning™ and creating exceptional training programmes. And thanks to a very special lady, Penny Perry for her continued support, sharing her insights and seeing what others cannot see.

Thanks to all those who have edited parts or the whole manuscript, especially Richard Ryan, Paris Beck, Arwen Meertens, Uschi Weinberge and Julia Merritt.

Finally, my husband who not only read and commented on drafts, but challenged my thinking. His support throughout the project has proven invaluable.

Finally, I am indebted to those I have met, whose names have been changed in this book, for providing such valuable information about their own experiences. They are always pleased to be helping others in this way.

Contents

Preface – Drawing the Map

There are few greater pleasures in the world than seeing a young person's face light up as they change their experience with, for example, reading, spelling, concentration and arithmetic. They suddenly exude a quiet confidence, as they organise their thoughts and begin feeling better about themselves. Their smiles are quite infectious.

This is my daily experience; I simply want to share it with you so we can help young people and adults start valuing their natural skills. It is merely a matter of helping them realise how best they learn and then teaching them how to use their new-found skills most effectively. I will give you a variety of examples here, there are many more, further into the book.

Once at a local book signing, Henry walked up to me to ask about spelling. I checked his mental images, and they were so close to his face they were on the end of his nose. He couldn't see the beginning nor end of any word. I asked him to visualise on my hand and gently walked backwards to about 6 feet. His face lit up, he thanked me and rushed off to tell his school friend.

I told William about this client, and it immediately resonated with him because he used to have words all around him, like on the inside of a crash helmet, which was exactly what he remembered seeing. He had been able to visualise small words well when he was very young, and, as he got older and the words become longer, he lost the beginning, end, top and bottom of the word – as if looking at a cut-out of just the centre of the word.

This book is primarily for parents, who are interested to discover how their children learn and think visually. In today's highly visual world, many children have quite exceptional skills that do not match the auditory way the school curriculum is delivered. Some children may have been diagnosed or maybe waiting for a diagnosis of a specific learning difficulty. However, mental imagery is just as applicable to all children, even those not considered to have a particular special educational need, and some maybe working at a lower level than their peers. Now everyone can find their hidden talents. This book will help every child succeed. Parents may recognise their children's strengths but don't know how to convert them into useful strategies for learning different topics, including many academic skills. These parents, with little time or resources, want to help their young people to achieve their potential. If you are the parent of a bright, creative child and no one has mentioned **mental imagery** to you, take a deep breath, the system has let you down. Here is your opportunity, to find out more – not merely a diagnosis, but a set of skills for you and your child to learn, and anyone can master them.

The book is also for open-minded teachers, educational professionals, psychologists and support staff who are looking for answers to the challenges they see children facing. Teachers will be delighted to find new skills enabling them to harness the natural strengths of their students and thus ensure bright creative children aren't left behind by the school system. They can integrate these skills into their classrooms, to help **all** their pupils achieve success, and to make the biggest impact with the time and resources available. Medical practitioners, curious about these skills, can extend the limited options they have available to help families. Instruction in mental-imagery skills can, especially in the formative years of a child, be literally life-changing.

This book is also for scholars looking for new avenues of specialist research in the world of learning differences.

The current learning pedagogy includes multi-sensory teaching and learning but does not explicitly cover how students learn through mental imagery. In elite sports, imagery has been used for decades.

Although those most at risk often have exceptional creative skills, many have not learned how to control their mental images in order to make learning easier. Visual learning skills can be taught in primary school and even before, to enable all young children to avoid a litany of pitfalls, including poor literacy, poor numeracy, poor concentration, sensory overload, fear, anxiety and even many mental health issues.

> Eric was 12 years old in a special needs school, and he had a large picture of his favourite Arsenal football player on his folder that he carried everywhere with him, so he was very familiar with the picture. I simply turned the folder over and asked if he could tell me what was on the cover. I looked at his eyes, and he was squinting, from behind his glasses far over into the distance. I asked him what he was doing, and he had no idea. I suggested he might like to bring the picture nearer, onto the window. I saw him rock back in surprise as he saw it on the window and could explain in perfect detail exactly what the player looked like and was wearing.

> I was getting on well chatting with Alistair, and I asked him if he could picture a lion. Before I could ask if it were male or female, he was off his chair and hiding behind it. I caught hold of the imaginary lion's chain and led him away from the little boy. His stress dropped, and he returned to sitting on his chair. On careful checking with other non-frightening objects, I discovered that all his pictures were literally on the end of his nose. He developed the skill to move them around to the best place for him. Pictures this close will cause a constant distraction for the student and present ADHD like symptoms.

It is well-known and documented that human innovation of all kinds – artistic, scientific, sporting, entrepreneurial, design, etc. – is driven by people who are not thinking the same way everyone before them has thought. Openness to new ideas and the originality of thought that create novel ways of thinking, most often come from people who are picturing what others do not see and making connections others ignore. This book explores these exceptional strengths from the viewpoint of an experienced coach practitioner, looking behind how people do what they do, and finding those exceptional strengths that are so often born out of excellent mental images. Having explored the strengths and weaknesses of older students, it has become apparent how to assist young children even before school age.

What others have failed to see are the flipsides of these strengths. Control of mental images is essential to avoid confusion and prevent those students from being overwhelmed by the current standardised teaching paradigm.

Moreover, highly visual learners often struggle to reach fluent literacy and numeracy skills.

I observed a classroom one day where John, a 10-year-old was causing havoc. He had this habit of shouting out "poodles" from time to time, accidentally encouraging others to do the same and then barking quite often broke out, as well! I unobtrusively watched the child whom you could see desperately wanted to do something, well anything, rather than listen to the teacher (according to the teacher) – talking, drawing, moving, etc. You could see his energy mounting, and sure enough, when it got too much he started shouting "poodles." The teacher then insisted that he look at her which raised his stress levels further. She gave him some paper with large squares on it. He started to draw manically, but the squares were not really a match for his big-picture thinking. However, drawing did calm him slightly, but he still wanted to talk about his pictures to the rest of the table. I had seen enough; I started to calm the environment in the classroom and focused on him, every time I saw his agitation increase. Every time he subsided before he started to shout out poodles. I discussed the situation with his headteacher, teacher and a lady who gave 1-1 support to an autistic child in the same class, I had taught two weeks before. Since then every morning her student walks in, sits down, spends a few seconds grounding and clearly loves the experience. In just a few days John had learned to control his own energy, to interact with other people's energy and develop a fabulous skill for life.

This book explains why and how the educational pedagogy, especially in the English-speaking countries, needs to be updated to include the teaching of mental imagery, starting with the youngest children. It also offers a method for repairing the confusion of older students, although neuroscience tells us that the younger the better. This two-pronged attack will stop the chaos from developing at its source with primary students as well as offering older students, who are wallowing in support for identified learning difficulties, a lifeline that is very easy for highly visual learners.

Most approaches to learning difficulties see everything as a deficit, a problem that should, but at the same time often can't be, fixed. Consequently, much of the research follows this same deficit model. I have taken the opposite approach: People with learning difficulties are simply learning differently, and it is for us to respect these individuals and understand how we can best teach them, in a manner that matches their preferred way of learning. **Learning differences shouldn't mean that you develop learning difficulties.** We should be harnessing the excellent skills, which these same people possess in disproportionate numbers, to help them with their challenges and make their learning experience more natural.

My approach is that of a practitioner; I don't seek to prove or justify my observations and the actions I have taken. Knowing what works, based on thousands of interventions, is good enough for me. I am not seeking to fix students; instead, I am providing them with options and a greater understanding of their current learning processes. I am working with people as individuals who need person-centred approaches, tailored to their particular challenges. Other trained practitioners and I have collected masses of anecdotal evidence, some of which we share anonymously in this book to illustrate learning points. I am not involved in formal research with a large number of students but would be happy to help others who want to research specific aspects of the work I have published. Most people now believe that there is a broad spectrum of how people learn. As a result, to collect meaningful data, you have to be very specific about the theme you are measuring – "one size does not fit all." You can't force change; however well-meaning parents are. For those who are desperate for a non-academic career this is always their choice.

Although the book refers to students, they can be any age from younger than 2 to older than 80. Similar skills can be offered to assist all of them. Interviewing and reading about successful adults, who have had learning challenges, has yielded more valuable insights. Then turning to our young clients, you can see the same themes developing in them, even in pre-school children. I have always worked as an outsider, without specialist training in education or an official professional position from which to explain or defend and shape my perspectives. I focus on primary research relying on stories, anecdotes, first-person accounts and my own experiences to help me develop this approach. I listen to affected students; they are the experts, and without their valuable assistance, these insights would not have been possible. I have come to trust them more than I do the conventional academic theories.

My observations and experiences have enabled me to develop techniques that complement conventional approaches. My methods empower the individual to take action, using resources they already possess, to positively affect any learning challenges and indeed their health. Above all, I needed to make teaching these essential skills person-centred, and thus easy for both the student and the teacher. I often talk directly to the audience, urging readers to try out their own experiences before teaching others.

This book may turn learning difficulties upside down; I hope you will be open to the challenges and the joy of success. Students need teachers to change the way they teach to include the way the brightest children learn.

In the words of Ralph Waldo Emerson, "Whatever course you decide upon, there is always someone to tell you that you are wrong. There are always difficulties arising which tempt you to believe that your critics are right. To map out a course of action and follow it to an end requires courage."

To summarise, this book will help you to enable all students, their parents and teachers to become expert in:

- Helping our talented creative young people excel.
- Understanding learning differences from the perspective of the person involved.
- Engaging people with their own experiences and seeing how simple tools can often create rapid change.
- Engaging families; the experts who know their children are bright and who want to be able to help them to learn more effectively.

- Assisting families to reduce their stress in the most challenging of circumstances.
- Changing a "common injustice," which results in those exceptional human beings, who just learn differently, being labelled deficient.
- Seeing how many of the challenging symptoms of learning differences can be prevented.

The Elephants in the Classroom is a natural companion and sequel to *Bridges to Success*. Both books support each other and build on common principles. This book is unique in that it delves deeper into understanding precisely what can go wrong when we don't introduce youngsters to their natural mental imagery and how this shortcoming contributes to all specific learning difficulties. It explains how their strengths manifest themselves in the classroom as deficits. This book also probes deeper in an effort to discover skills for reducing dyslexia, and dyscalculia, then deeper still for dyspraxia, ADHD, Asperger's and autism. My focus has been to understand the role of mental imagery in learning differences, and thus enabling all students to excel. Since publishing *Bridges to Success* in 2011, I have learned even more about the key role mental images play across all learning differences.

I pride myself on writing books that introduce new concepts in a way that anyone can understand – you won't need any previous skills. This book includes NeuroLinguistic Programming (NLP), Energetic NLP[1], Thought Pattern Management[2], breathing techniques and other processes; providing you with all the tools and information you will need.

In short, this book has the potential to change the lives of hundreds of thousands of students. It is, I believe, unique. It is an in-depth study of **why** it is crucial for students to understand their mental images, **how** these images affect their abilities to think and learn, who these perspectives are most likely to affect and **when** it is best to take action and with **which** skills.

These are some of our most talented students; we need to get them out of special education classes and let the universe benefit from their new ideas. A lack of knowledge about how students learn visually contributes to all learning difficulties.

Everyone knows a bright child who is being left behind, so please pass this book along to their parents.

Every Child CAN Succeed.   Olive Hickmott, 2019

How to use this book

As this book is about mental imagery, you will see:

- Illustrations on most pages to help you create your own images and to get a flavour of how creative, imaginative students learn. They are deliberately not perfect, to encourage others to develop their skills; anyone can improve his skills.
- There are also many stories and mini-examples of students' experiences to illustrate various points. You will learn how students have simply had life-changing experiences when they are open to learning simple new skills. These experiences are often unique to the individual, but they are built on certain common themes. The reason for telling you of other people's paths is to inspire you with possibilities for you or your student's particular circumstance. Students are referred to as he, just for simplicity, nothing is gender specific.
- The examples can also highlight the obstacles, blocks and frustrations many people experience, which is all quite normal, and if you need additional assistance, we are here to help you.
- Throughout this book, you will find suggestions of other resources to help you. Whenever possible, I point to other books, including *Bridges to Success*, websites and videos that you may find useful, acknowledging the sources that have influenced this book. This book is also part of a more extensive programme, see details at www.empoweringlearning.co.uk, where we offer you continued support, resources, videos, etc. for your particular needs and share the vast bank of tips and tricks that make such a difference to our students. Don't be afraid to ask! Much of the material is free, and there is a subscription programme for those who want to journey deeper yet and change the paradigm for these students.
- You will also find in the book some of my favourite quotes that have meant so much to me and this work.

1.
Getting started – Mental Imagery

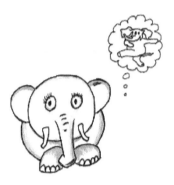

This book contains a number of vital messages for children, parents, teachers, schools, colleges and governments.

Mental Imagery, the basis of visual learning, is the key to many different aspects of education. Remember mental imagery is a thinking and learning tool for every child; some have good skills; some have exceptional skills.

Explicitly incorporating this style of learning in education will:

- enable students to learn in the most effective way for them
- facilitate a shift from a deficit frame to an increased awareness of students' strengths
- reduce learning difficulties.

Note: I trust you have read the preface before coming here, as it gives valuable insights you will need before progressing further.

Why I Wrote this book?

I have a message that affects every child, especially those struggling with literacy, numeracy, concentration as well as diagnosed or undiagnosed learning difficulties. **"You have great natural skills, and there is more than one way to learn to spell, read, and concentrate."**

I have a message for every parent whose child has been awaiting assessment for months and years, because of our overloaded educational services. **"Read this book and start helping your child develop new skills, simply and easily, while awaiting a formal assessment."**

I have a message for every parent of a child thought to be on the autistic spectrum. **"There are simple skills to teach you and your child how to feel safe and not to be overwhelmed by the world and by the activity of your child's very fast, exceptional brain. They can learn in a way that best suits them; it's easy and fun."**

I have a message for every headteacher and school. **"Teaching mental imagery in the earlier years will reduce stress and the need for special education funding later. Challenge the current educational paradigm, and give yourself the freedom to teach in a way that works for every child in your class."**

I have a message for many adults who are often ashamed of their poor spelling and reading. **"Let go of the shame and guilt; you simply weren't taught in a way that worked for you. Don't be frightened, don't be scared, and don't blame yourself, your parents or your school. Just come on board, be curious and enjoy the journey."**

I have a message for businesses. **"It is clear that our society needs all the inventive minds available to solve the problems of the current world. People who think and learn differently can devise incredible business solutions, as acknowledged by GCHQ and Microsoft, for example."**

I have a message for governments: **"Mental imagery should be incorporated into teaching at primary school and before, to maximise the skills of these exceptionally talented children. Nobody wants students crushed by a society that sees only deficits and ignores their gifts; junior and senior school is too late to begin."**

I have a message for the whole education system including parents who have key roles: **"Our children are here to teach us there is another way of being and teaching those who are thinking and learning in neurodivergent ways. It isn't the same way we have been teaching for decades. The world is different now and these children know how best they learn."**

Since publishing *Bridges to Success* in 2011, I have learned more from my clients, made further discoveries and learned from related fields, such as neuroscience, metacognition, physical eyesight, brain plasticity, nutrition, the effects of trauma on learning and many others. Everything has come together to form a complete picture of how humans think and learn through mental imagery and how some adults and children don't understand how to make the best use of their, often exceptional, skills.

I had a choice to see what I was taught or to believe what I saw in my students; they are the experts. Anything is possible when you observe and hold a space for the students to explain their experiences. Sure enough, I saw things that the students and others wouldn't have believed possible for these "learning disabled" people, who aren't disabled at all. They just think and learn differently.

The education system needs to step back and see the bigger picture, which ironically is often a strength of these students.

There isn't one solution for everyone, but there are themes that are common to many. I am an expert in mental imagery and how this affects learning and thinking. For example, each of the following topics has a skill you can learn to improve visually:

- If reading is a problem, students may not have progressed from *sounds* of words to *images* of the word for rapid recognition.
- Anxiety is going to affect our gut, and that affects our brain and can destroy memory.
- Regularly zoning-out may be a sign of sensory overload from outside stimuli or our own internal images.
- Shying away from being touched indicates being ungrounded.

These are just a few of the topics that will benefit every parent, teacher, adult and child, not only to reduce learning difficulties dramatically but to make everyone's experience better by focusing on their ignored visual strengths.

If you have already read **Bridges to Success**, you will be familiar with some of the content and the great tools offered there. This book digs deeper into all aspects of mental imagery. It provides the reader with a unique **new perspective** on the contribution of mental images, to the whole spectrum of dyslexia, dyscalculia, dysgraphia, dyspraxia, ADHD, Asperger's, autism, sensory overload, OCD, 48XXYY and many others. Very different experiences of mental imagery characterise learning differences. In short, mental imagery is a missing key to understanding both exceptional strengths and their associated challenges. It is one of **The Elephants in the Classroom.**

I hope I will inspire you to share my passion for these topics because this is happening to the brightest students. You will all know many. If I have any expertise (and the more we learn, the more we realise how ignorant we are), it is a skill for connecting a whole host of related subjects. You will read about mental imagery, neuroscience, metacognition, stress, trauma, anxiety, seeing behind the obvious, connecting with the bigger picture, individual strengths, the education system, energy, mental health, personal development tools and human rights. I and my trained practitioners, have a growing knowledge base and offer this unique approach because we refuse to be limited by current paradigms.

I can best describe myself as a Forensic Learning Coach, unravelling how people think and learn, and discovering what works best for them.

What are Mental Images?

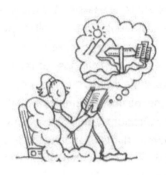

People often ask what mental images are, and here is a simple explanation. Mental imagery is normal, just like breathing, and is quite simply the images we hold in our head. All these images, presented as either pictures or videos, are held in our occipital lobe, the part of our brain just above the "dent" at the top of our neck where the skull meets the spine.

We use mental images every minute of every day, often outside of our conscious awareness, but we seldom know how to make the best use of them. For example, how do you find things like your house or your car? How do you recognise people you know; your spouse, parents or children? How do you locate the ingredients for a meal? How do you plan what to wear and where to find your clothes? People take mental images for granted yet know next to nothing about them.

My own practice and the work of other Empowering Learning™ Practitioners has helped me piece together the vital role of mental imagery in the whole learning process. **The power of pictures.**

The Elephants in the Classroom

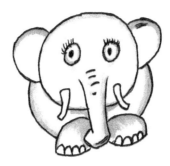

The expression the "Elephant in the Room" is an idiom used to describe a big important issue or obvious fact that everyone is aware of but isn't discussed, as such a discussion is considered to be uncomfortable.

The role of mental imagery is just that. Mental imagery is a vital part of learning, but very few people ever acknowledge or discuss it. There can be many reasons for this, for example:

- It is such a natural skill for many that they have no idea that others may not be equally blessed.
- People may feel that they don't have strong mental images.
- People don't realise the connections between mental imagery and learning differences.

This book is dedicated to the role of mental imagery in learning. It will help every parent and child to understand how mental imagery contributes to the learning process, from a child's earliest days and certainly before they reach school age.

As you go through the book you will find other associated **Elephants in the Classroom,** such as safety, strengths, grounding, controlling mental images and other academic skills that are supported by mental images.

What is meant by Neurodiversity?

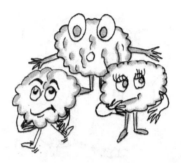

"Neurodiversity" came into our language several years ago. The human population is understood to be a neurodiverse group with some people learning and thinking in a **neurotypical** way that matches the way schools teach students. Others are thinking and learning in **neurodivergent** ways that do not match the way they are being taught in school[3]; unfortunately, these students often display dyslexic, dyscalculic, dyspraxic, ADHD, Asperger's and autistic symptoms.

Increasingly, people realise that these young people and adults learn differently but they don't know how to ensure that the skills they are using work effectively. This book is not only relevant for students, who are learning and thinking in neurodivergent ways, but it is also beneficial for all learners and their families to understand more about how we learn effectively.

History tells us that many great inventions and a great deal of the progress that humanity has achieved thus far has been made by exceptional people, who have not fitted into a neurotypical model and were often ostracised by the education system of the day.

But now, with the benefits of neuroscience, we have not only the information but the skills, to enable us to teach in a way that works for neurodivergent learners.

Everyone has Strengths

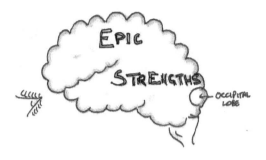

Everyone has strengths and learns most easily by employing those assets. Some people have genuinely exceptional strengths (see Chapter 6) that you may have dismissed and teaching those individuals how to use these strengths to make learning and thinking more effective will completely transform them from debilitating symptoms to perceived advantages.

These same students can be **E**xceptionally **P**erceptive, **I**maginative and **C**reative; in short, they are **EPIC**. All of our students are EPIC and have neurodivergent thinking and learning skills. In studying children and adults with exceptional strengths, we have explored how they do what they do well. The vast majority have fabulous mental imagery stored in their occipital lobe. Using mental images just for pictures means that teachers and students don't value them for literacy, numeracy and so many other academic skills.

In this book, we are not going to distinguish between various learning differences while examining the fundamental skills and challenges of these EPIC students. We not only acknowledge the enormous strengths of neurodiversity in our students but provide you with the skills to explore and enhance these strengths while determining how best to employ them – their **Misunderstood Greatness**

THE PROBLEMS

This section examines the problem, where things are going wrong for our EPIC students, as well as their families and their teachers. We look at the contributions of various educational assessments and connect the dots to unexplored mental imagery.

I regularly speak to parents who explain their child has been diagnosed as have dyslexia, ADHD, a spot of Asperger's, etc. My immediate reaction is: "How can this long list be right? There must be a connection between them?" We will explore one of the connections that is simple and yet inordinately powerful: **Mental imagery is a vital part of all learning.**

Bright Kids are Left Behind

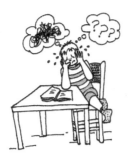

Sadly, many bright students are unnecessarily being left behind or worse. Some come to believe they are stupid; as a result, they may get bullied just for being different. A child who grows up surrounded by such misery can experience trauma, self-loathing and in exceptional circumstances, attempt suicide.

We all know bright students who have been left behind, struggling with a mass of diagnosed or undiagnosed learning difficulties. Evidence indicates these people are just learning differently. However, with everyone focused on telling them what they can't do, pointing out the student's deficits, putting these students into a box of "being faulty," they will naturally lose sight of their tremendous strengths. The current paradigm conveniently ignores such strengths, and the parents of these students are left to advocate for adjustments in their education, such as extra time, time out of class and using computers.

I believe it is our responsibility to find ways to teach these EPIC students in a way that matches their strengths. Bringing mental imagery into the pedagogy will free up the students' creative brains and dramatically improve a broad range of skills from literacy to concentration. Not teaching to these strengths is a critical shortcoming that will be illustrated in real stories of students who don't necessarily follow the "textbook" approach to learning.

A Parent's Heartache

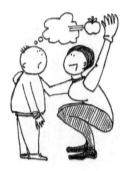

Trying to help children who learn differently – both to you, as a parent, and to the average child in their class – can be an enormous heartache and source of frustration for both parents and teachers. My heart goes out to all those parents I meet who have no idea how and why their children are struggling so much and who have not even heard of "mental imagery."

As parents strive to do the very best for their children, they encounter various question on social media such as:
"I am new to dyslexia; what do I do now?"
"My child is struggling; at what age should I press for a diagnosis?"
"I can see my child facing the same challenges I did, and I feel so guilty."
"Whom do I need to contact to make some real progress?"

To those, I say: **"Learning differently doesn't mean you have learning difficulties. We can empower you with new knowledge and skills."**

Let's assume just for a moment that there is nothing wrong with these EPIC students; there is no condition to assess, no "deficit" to find; only their neurodivergent strengths and how best to use them. Perhaps the questions we should be asking are: How we can best teach a neurodivergent population? Or: How can we change the way we teach to include our brightest children? These questions were first poised in 1911 by Hans

Asperger who "instead of seeing the children in his care as flawed, broken, or sick, believed they were suffering from neglect by a culture that had failed to provide them with the teaching methods suited to their individual style of learning. He had an uncanny knack for spotting signs of potential in every boy or girl, no matter how difficult or rebellious they were alleged to be." We must urgently address this fundamental question that has largely been overlooked, since that time. We need vital help from students, parents and teachers to bring about change.

Working as a family is essential to success. You will learn how you can best investigate your children's skills even before they go to school and indeed before they learn to talk. Curiosity encourages the development of a healthy, mutual learning environment where students feel empowered to grow. Moreover, this allows whole families to learn and grow together. When students learn a new strategy, they have to practice to become an expert. Any new skill you are developing requires practice. In some instances, however, young people may choose not to do this for a variety of reasons. Although they do not want to fail again, they may also not want to let down or show up friends or other family members, who share the same challenge. When working with students, I ask them to identify who else they can now teach, to reinforce the learning and encourage people to help each other.

The ability to successfully learn new skills is fundamental to the existence of every living creature. As we grow up, we continually acquire new talents naturally, often with little education. Parents of EPIC students often marvel at how their child knows about things nobody has taught them. However, their natural capabilities can pull them in a different direction where traditional learning poses a much tougher challenge. When EPIC students don't naturally acquire these required skills and conventions, the world becomes more confusing, and they may often be identified as being "learning disabled." I have lost count of how many parents, who, after a short explanation of mental imagery, exclaim: "**This makes so much sense**".

The Teachers' Challenge

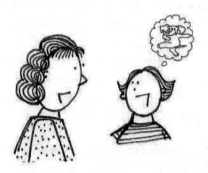

Schools are hectic environments, with large class sizes and very limited resources. Mandated standards and government statistics measure the schools and their students. Learning differences create extra work and teachers are often bewildered as to why some students encounter so many difficulties. Teaching students about mental images creates a more natural learning experience for the students and their teachers.

Teachers need to learn about the vital role that mental images play in the visual learning process. They can be equipped with simple methods to check their students' skills and suggest strategies to improve them. Mental imagery is a hidden skill, but a few simple questions will shine a light on the students' experiences. Identifying their natural skills and mental imagery capabilities can be easily detected even in nursery or pre-school.

This book will provide every teacher with new skills that only take minutes to learn and use. For example, if a student is asked to picture an elephant, and he describes a blue elephant with pink spots, believe him and use this to develop his skills further. Ask for further details, like the size of their ears, what is the elephant doing – get the student to explain the whole picture – this is how we introduce young children to their own mental images, and it is straightforward.

Diagnosis and Assessment

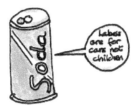

Diagnosis and assessment drive the current paradigm, where students attempt various tests, and the results indicate deficits which are diagnosed as dyslexia, ADHD, etc. In recent years more and more learning struggles have been identified as Specific Learning Difficulties (SpLD). Such diagnoses or "labels," as many people refer to them, have both positive and negative aspects. In many respects, labels serve as shorthand for the range of challenges a student is facing, helping people understand more about his condition and to provide him with extra support. The downside is that labels are limiting, keep students pigeonholed, and fail to recognise their strengths, skills and tenacity to succeed, especially when the word "lifelong" is included. All this contributes to a feeling of disempowerment that discourages EPIC students, their parents and teachers from taking advantage of any opportunities to improve.

In addition, there is a well-known expression, "When you have met one student with say autism, you have met only one student." Obviously not all students share the same symptoms. For example, one may not be able to focus on exams; another may love the silence in exams; one may be able to read avidly; another may forget instantly what he has read. At Empowering Learning™, we focus on the skills someone wants to learn, not the labels they have attached. This approach offers a functional breakdown, tailored to the individual, which avoids some of the downsides of focusing on generic labels. To best help struggling students, identify the specific function they find difficult, find the root cause and work from there – I refer to this as **functional learning**. In the same way medics are exploring functional medicine[4] and neurologists are exploring functional neurology[5]. You will see in Chapter 5 references to the very different ways students experience mental images and in Chapter 6 lists of possible symptoms that often are rooted in a common cause, and I can assure you that individuals only have a few of them.

Assessments almost always fail to consider mental imagery and only pay lip service to strengths, usually mentioning them as a "non-negative," e.g. not reversing letters, for dyslexics. However, the skills that lie behind their strengths are ignored and missing from all standard assessments.

By contrast, we should be addressing the exceptional strengths these EPIC students have and looking behind their strengths to discover **"how they do what they do"** and how can students re-use these skills elsewhere to overcome challenges.

Relationship to Learning Difficulties

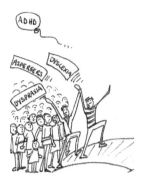

Creating mental images can be both very impressive and yet often quite overwhelming. EPIC students often possess a fast, hyperactive mind that will have a huge impact on their ability to function. These mental images are the source of many genius-level abilities. However if they spiral out of control for a small child, it can lead to years of confusion and even withdrawal from the world. At best, they can be very distracting, and a child can be caught up in his own images that pop up, unexpectedly outside of any conscious control.

> Six-year-old Freddy was asked to picture an elephant. Freddy, with a neurodivergent thinking style and an inability to concentrate, told me about six elephants, all different colours which were ninja dancing. His sister had a much more neurotypical style had just one grey elephant.

At worst, EPIC students may not be able to have any control over the number of pictures or select whether they are still or moving. Image control is something that can be taught in school and also pre-school to avoid some of the overload that those very young children experience and which causes them to shut down. This is the silent **Elephant in the Classroom**.

So, let's have a look at what is happening when we haven't learned how to control our mental images.

The thing to notice here is the contribution mental imagery plays in many learning difficulties/differences. Because mental images are not seen nor explored and quite often ignored, these connections are virtually unknown - they represent one of the **Elephants in the Classroom.**

Diagnosis	Unrecognised mental imagery symptoms
Poor literacy, Dyslexia, Dysgraphia	Not picturing still letters/words.
Poor numeracy, Dyscalculia	Not picturing still numbers.
ADHD	Too many screens, too near, distractions, etc.
Dyspraxia	Can't control their images.
Asperger's, Sensory Overload, 48XXYY[6] and Autism	Cascades of mental images with no structure causing anxiety. Visual recall can be excellent, while visual construct can be frightening.
Hyperlexia[7]	Obsession with the way a word sounds, with no understanding of its meaning.
OCD traits	Repeated actions that have not been captured visually, e.g. locking the door

If mental imagery for words and numbers is not taught explicitly, about 50% of the population (measurement taken at Empowering Learning™ workshops), will not naturally develop these skills. Thus, it is left to chance.

Without mental imagery, many creative career paths are blocked, for example, such as design, engineering and the media.

On an even more serious note, many of the symptoms of out-of-control mental images can often spill over into mental health issues, for example, depression and withdrawal.

Chapter 6 has more details about how these invisible skills go wrong.

Energy and Grounding

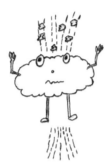

Another problem with Coke cans is that when they are shaken enough, they tend to explode when opened. This can happen with our students as well. After a long day in school, they may be ready to explode at home.

Sometimes the day in school may have seemingly gone well, but on other occasions, there may have been problems, that built up inside your student to the point of explosion. This energy build-up is very common with ungrounded sensitive students.

Being grounded might be understood as feeling balanced and collected, leading to wiser decisions, feeling more focused and being more present with those around us. We can feel most grounded when we are well-rested and in a comfortable environment.

Being ungrounded can be the cause of oversensitivity and feeling vulnerable in everyday situations. Just like a tree with unearthed roots or a building without firm foundations, a person who is ungrounded is more likely to be affected by the events that happen around them.

When it comes to dealing with new experiences, and school can be a unique experience every day, being able to stay calm and grounded with time to process all this further information afterwards in a quiet environment is invaluable. Without this space, processing new information is often an explosion of thoughts, frequently visual, that vie for your attention.

Please note that being grounded in this context is feeling fully in your body, embodied. This is nothing the same as grounding a child by sending them to their bedroom in disgrace, although it would be useful to get grounded in this situation too.

There are many references in this book to energy and grounding so you will learn more to assist you and your student – another **Elephant in the Classroom** that is closely related to feeling safe.

KEY CONCEPTS

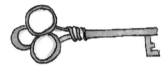

Before going further, I need to introduce you to some key concepts and terminology. Readers may be familiar with the names of various diagnoses but know little more. I will present some key concepts in a straightforward manner – such concepts have been fundamental to our approach.

- What is meant by metacognition?
- The contribution made by neuroscience.
- Big Picture Visual Thinkers.
- The Educational Pedagogy.

What is Meant by Metacognition?

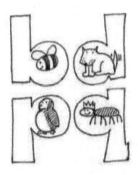

Metacognition directly answers the question "How do people do what they do?" Metacognition provides an awareness and understanding of one's thought processes. Using metacognition, we can unpack how people succeed, identifying their strategies and teaching those skills to others who may find it more difficult. These improvements are the basis of a growth mindset, enabling us to excel in any chosen field, by learning from the best.

Understanding a student's confusion and how this all develops opens up an opportunity for early prevention. Working with a vast range of clients over the last 15 years, from four to eighty-five years of age, I have been privileged to gain insights into how some people are successful and how others are plagued by confusion that deepens with time. I have studied successful entrepreneurs, marketers, artists and copywriters as well as young children who have no idea how to spell and read, and watch helplessly as their classmates find literacy so easy. The underlying pattern is similar: **The effective use of mental imagery**. For example, what starts as simple letter reversals (a four-year-old not knowing the difference between p, q, b and d) can develop into them seeing whole words moving on the page, escalating into hundreds of mental images and resulting in nausea. As we might expect, the young person's behaviour will, not surprisingly, often deteriorate.

A Contribution from Neuroscience

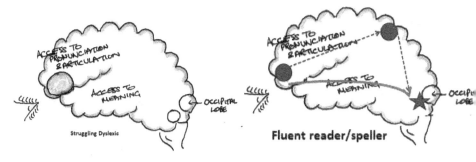

Visualising words has been researched as far back as 1963 by L. D. Radaker[8], but since then, there seems to have been people who just refused to believe the experiences that students described. What is more, nobody else has recognised how visual skills dramatically contribute to the broader field of learning. Hence, they were not put into educational settings. In sports it is just the opposite – some coaches and many elite athletes have used mental imagery for decades.

Neuroscience is continually evolving[9] and has offered us some vital information which, you will see in this book, starting in the area of how mental imagery is essential for fluent literacy. The diagrams above are the basis of our first discoveries into teaching literacy. Consider a struggling dyslexic, who is trying to process every word in the front of his brain while the other diagram shows the brain activity of a non-dyslexic, where words pass into the Word Form Area (adjacent to the occipital lobe) at the back of the brain. The Word Form Area connects word images with pronunciation, articulation and meaning to achieve fluent reading and spelling. Brain scanning techniques enabled us to learn from neuroscientists about these differences and thus develop targeted teaching.

Big Picture Visual Thinkers

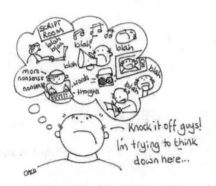

EPIC students are often big-picture thinkers, permanently curious, always wanting to know why, with their heads full of amazing mental images. For example, to picture a giraffe, a big picture thinker may think of a whole herd of giraffes roaming across the savanna, with a multitude of other animals. Also known as visual-spatial intelligence, this occurs when students possess the ability to visualise the picture accurately and modify their surroundings based on their perceptions.

Unfortunately, lack of control of their mental images can lead to confusion, anxiety, internal chaos, closing down and even withdrawal from the world. The latter is the last thing we want for these EPIC students, who have such great talents to offer us.

If EPIC students manage to avoid this confusion, they develop creative and imaginative skills, which are rooted in their ability to create and use mental images in all sorts of areas of their lives, including art, design, sports and entrepreneurship.

The Educational Pedagogy

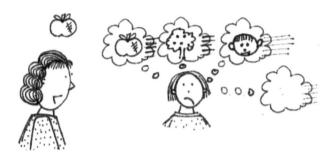

And finally, pedagogy is the discipline that deals with the theory and practice of teaching. Pedagogy informs all aspects of teaching – strategies, actions, judgments and decisions – by taking into consideration various theories of learning, understanding students' needs, and their backgrounds and the interests of individual students. Teaching typically includes showing students visual images, pictures, graphs etc. and makes no mention at all of the images students created in their heads, which may or may not be accurate – this is their visual learning skill and teachers should incorporate it into the current education pedagogy.

We certainly don't want to throw out phonics; it is most valuable especially for words you have never seen before; however, I would like the educational curriculum/system to explicitly include mental imagery in order to accelerate learning, especially for EPIC students in order to minimise stress with literacy and numeracy.

Mental imagery is the specialist subject of EPIC students. My experience is that hitherto struggling students suddenly look at their teacher or parent and say: "I can do this; it's easy."

THE SOLUTIONS

To find solutions to these problems the rest of this book will look at and expand on the following areas:

Chapter 2: My Personal Story: Growing up in the dark – How my own dyslexic, ADHD and Asperger's symptoms underpinned my passion for embracing learning differences and minimising the attendant confusion and stress. The chapter finishes with some of the people who have inspired me to believe that anything is possible with an open mind. A full list of further reading can be found at the back of this book.

Chapter 3: Exceptional Strengths of EPIC Students – A celebration of visual learning, exploring the excellent skills that students possess and their underlying talents.

Chapter 4: Teachers Teach, Learners Learn – The real differences between teaching practices and the obstacles that discourage effective learning. Metacognition has helped to break down learning differences into their visual elements and how with a growth mindset, students can further develop their exceptional skills.

Chapter 5: A New Perspective: Mysteries, Contradictions and Updating the Paradigm – The paradox of things that seem illogical until we look for solutions through the lens of mental imagery. Anyone can adjust or modify the current paradigm by:

- Following a simple 7-step process
- Exploring with students their underlying visual experiences.

Chapter 6: When Mental Imagery Goes Wrong – This chapter explains the challenges we see with students who have not learned how best to use mental imagery.

Chapter 7: Freeing Trapped Potential – This chapter really connects the dots, explaining how the students can use their innate visual skills to help them excel in other areas. It offers specific examples of how to improve handwriting, increase concentration, reduce anxiety, improve reading and spelling, improve sleep, diminish sensory overload and increase resilience. All of these contribute to improving behaviour.

Conclusion: Creating your own Map – The simple steps anyone can take, to help those struggling with the challenges of learning differences. We have a whole class plan for the youngest students and simple remedial actions for older students.

Mental imagery can unblock neurodivergent children's thinking and learning challenges.

2.
My Personal Story: Growing up in the Dark

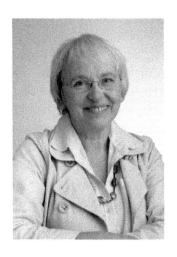

My real passion is to alleviate and prevent much of the confusion that threatens to overwhelm EPIC students. Teachers and parents of children under 7 years old need to incorporate visualisation into any and all forms of teaching, especially literacy and numeracy. Nobody showed me how to use my visual brain for literacy – something that has affected my entire life. **Would have been simply turning on what had been turned off.**

Allow me the indulgence of sharing my own story in this regard.

A Reformed Dyslexic

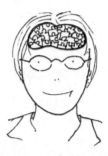

I call myself a reformed dyslexic, because I struggled in school with literacy, long before dyslexia was commonly understood in schools. Had I been born later, I would probably have been labelled dyslexic. I have subsequently learned for myself those vital missing skills that have in turn inspired my efforts to help others. My hyperactive brain could have also got me diagnosed with ADHD and a splash of Asperger's. I am now an avid reader which has helped me to learn and reduce any number of other symptoms. My curiosity prompted me to discover why some EPIC students are successful while others struggle. From my perspective, there are very different experiences of mental imagery that dramatically affect every learner.

I live in a permanent state of curiosity, with a 'jigsaw-puzzle' brain that people around me might find challenging but which has, I believe, the potential to be quite powerful. My mind can make intuitive leaps and see connections in things that others may keep separate. I see things clearly that others do not see. Things are obvious to me – I don't know why – perhaps because of fast connections, insights or something else. There is nothing special about me, my brain likes understanding 'why' and connect things, like huge jigsaw puzzles, in several dimensions. I see the same skills in many of my students. For someone who is neurodivergent, the biggest challenge is to present this knowledge in a way others can cope with and take action.

School – Trying to Learn in the Dark

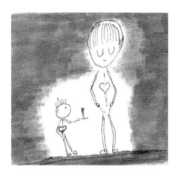

Entering the school system, in the UK, at age 4, my literacy was progressing, fitfully. By the age of seven, I was really struggling. My report at 16 says: "Hampered by lack of vocabulary and atrocious spelling, she has an inability to express herself clearly. It really would help if Olive could learn to spell." I had been in the same school for 12 years and was generally a good but often shy student. It took me another 40 years to discover the secret of why literacy, in English, seemed so tricky. Having no mental images of words was like trying to read and write in the dark. I realised then that schools take no responsibility for their teaching methods negatively affecting their students' ability to spell or read fluently. I was expected to fix this, and I had no idea how to do it. I now regret, missing out on all that fabulous children's literature, for I could read to myself, but I couldn't remember anything I read. As a result, I found reading boring, and I only read those things I had to, rather than for pleasure.

Also, I can remember, as if it were yesterday, with a clear picture of the room, being told I was tone-deaf and being told to leave the music class immediately. I was only around ten years old, and I was rejected without knowing why. How many EPIC students are moved down a set without any explanation? This feeling resonates with what many of our EPIC students experience today about literacy, numeracy and so many other subjects.

They can't do it, and they have no idea why. My spirits were kept up by excelling at sports and being good at maths, so maths is the degree I completed.

A teacher once told my mother that my brain was far too fast for my hand, which was nearly accurate. Whilst reading this book, you may notice I have a very different perspective on many things, which is a common and positive dyslexic trait. I have written this book to share these different approaches with students, their parents and their teachers.

I now feel privileged not to have been given any label in the past, although I knew my literacy skills were well below average. I recall wanting to disappear into the floor when we were reading aloud in class – dreading my turn coming around. I never read for pleasure until I was nearly 40 when I wanted to read to our son. How could I contemplate reading anything for fun when I found it such a nightmare? For me, it was extremely difficult to remember what I had read and, when putting a book down, a bookmark was essential. I also studied French for years and never managed to achieve 'O' level. Now, whose idea was it to teach me another language, when I couldn't spell in my first language?

However, I did GCSE and A Levels Maths a year early, which was almost unheard of in the 1970s, thanks partly to my excellent mental images of numbers. I then graduated from Sussex University with an honours degree in mathematics.

Just like my clients, I was the child who always asked "Why should we do this?" and "How does that work?" I have learned so much from clients, and come to understand more about what each brain wants and needs in order to make learning easier, and decipher what is happening for the student. I don't pretend to know all the answers for every learning difficulty as I am also continually learning, but I hope the understanding you will gain from this book will give you many new perspectives to try.

My Corporate Career

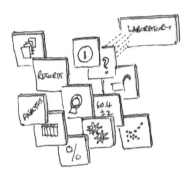

University was followed by a successful career as a software engineer, first developing systems for medical blood analysis which had 150 software programs all interacting with thousands of patient records. When looking for a software bug, I remember developing the strange knack of being almost able to dialogue with the programmes, asking which could have changed those data bits incorrectly – visualising the components in my head, trying them out and fixing what didn't work – all using clear mental images.

I progressed from engineer to department manager and finally research and development director in a hi-tech data communications company. I was involved in the early days of the Internet, managing up to 100 software engineers, hardware engineers, authors and a customer support staff. One of the excellent skills I possessed was to be able to see problems and challenges from very different perspectives; a useful skill when working in a complex global company. The downside, of course, is that you can be overwhelmed by seeing too many different perspectives to make a decision.

When, years later, I first discovered that good spellers could see words in their head, I was dumbfounded that I had never thought of trying this. I was furious that no one had told me about this skill, which others had taken for granted. I then turned this into a passion for offering others these skills.

Revisiting my own Education

Living in a permanent state of curiosity, I challenge the status quo and want to know why things are the way they are. A neuro-linguistic programming (NLP) training programme introduced me to visualising words in just 15 minutes. Those 15 minutes set me off on this new journey of discovery and ultimately changed my life. Picture visualisation works efficiently for most people, but many need to develop new skills for words and numbers. Having discovered how people who are good at spelling do it, I worked out a method to teach others to achieve the same exceptional success rates. I needed to help them resolve areas of confusion, such as letters jumping around on the page, being overwhelmed, stressed out or having low self-esteem, before they could all achieve what they wanted. Then I moved onto the rest of literacy, for example, reading, comprehension and handwriting. I even discovered how I made maths easy for myself when others struggled. Above all, I needed to make teaching these essential skills person-centred, easy for both the student and the teacher. My consulting practice, Empowering Learning,™ was born in 2002 and continues, today, to train people around the globe.

With a bit of help from inspirational authors like Temple Grandin's brilliant account of her own experiences, I figured out how to help students improve concentration while avoiding sensory overload, fidgeting, zoning-out and so many other impediments.

As is my wont, I looked outside the box to discover what neurodiversity, neuroscience and metacognition could contribute to the story and found limited but valuable research. For example, most people believe that everyone's symptoms are different, especially on the autistic spectrum. I agree with researchers that even with dyslexia, different people are affected to varying degrees. But exploring the bigger picture, including dyspraxia, dyscalculia, ADHD, Asperger's, 48XXYY and autism, I discovered a theme running through all of them and that theme is how we use mental imagery for thinking and learning. It is common to almost all neurodivergent skills and is, of course, the reason for this book.

As my journey continued, I realised I could now overcome some of the challenges I had assumed that I had no control over, and the process of change was really gratifying. I also realised that I had always been able to visualise numbers (hence the maths degree) but had never imagined visualising words.

What did I need from my teachers? I was great at mental arithmetic because I was easily visualising numbers and all I needed was a teacher who asked me how I did maths so quickly and who would then help me to learn how to add words to my pictures; **Unleashing trapped potential**. These skills would have prevented me from growing up riddled with anxiety and stress about literacy.

What I Realise Now

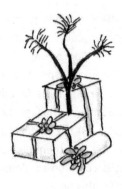

I realise now I had very fast-moving images of pictures, often moving so rapidly I couldn't recall them. I had no mental images of words and yet good mental images of numbers for mental arithmetic. As a result of learning how to use mental imagery for words, I let go of my crippling confusion over spelling and reading. I love reading now, whereas it used to send me to sleep and my spelling is patchy. The area I have never caught up with involves all the technical details of English, such as sentence construction, styles of writing, etc., all of which should have become embedded at a young age. I was too busy just trying to spell each word.

My story is like so many of those with whom I work – they have fabulous visual skills, neither they nor others appreciate. Nobody has taught them how to optimise these skills to visualise numbers, letters, whole words, sentences and stories; keeping them still or moving them at will and moving pictures around to see different perspectives. I am always distressed to meet so many adults who have been made to feel ashamed of their spelling and reading and are too traumatised even to discuss it.

After understanding how to help people explore their mental images and learning how to teach these simple skills, I moved onto really understanding how neurodivergent people use their mental images for all manner of different activities, often in situations far superior to my own experiences. I added brain research, personal energy, motivation to change, the concept of growth mind-sets and family coaching, all in an effort to facilitate learning.

I have seen time and time again, that if students are prepared to practice, as I have, to change a long-established habit, they can overcome the confusing and debilitating symptoms, in minutes or hours, thus escaping the trauma of failure.

I didn't value my visual skills as a child. Now I realise the gift I had been given – to see many different perspectives simultaneously and make extraordinary connections at high speed – was the very skill that made words so confusing, as they "flew past" in a blur. Like many other people, I had taken my positive skills for granted and not realised that it wasn't second nature to everyone. These skills are invaluable to me. I employ them many times, every day, especially when coaching individuals, to really understand another person's experience. I am now very appreciative of these valuable gifts and wouldn't be without them. All my clients have outstanding gifts, but they often don't realise their own exceptional and diverse skills.

I have always worked as an outsider, without specialist training in education or an official professional position from which to explain or defend and shape my perspectives. I have focused on primary research relying on stories, anecdotes, first-person accounts and my own experiences to help me develop this approach. I listen to affected EPIC students; they are the experts, and without their valuable assistance, these insights would not have been possible. I have come to trust them more than I do many conventional academic theories. My observations and experiences have enabled me to develop techniques that complement conventional approaches. As a result, I can empower individuals to take action, using resources they already possess in order to positively affect their health and offset any learning challenges.

Those Who Have Inspired Me

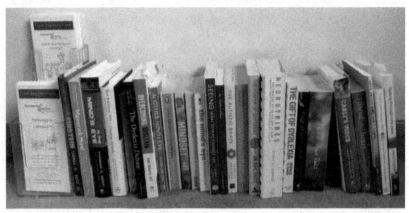

Many people believe it is time for a change. I believe we must find a way of implementing this change for our super-creative, imaginative students who are not coping well with the education system and whose talents are thus often minimized or overlooked entirely. Here I will paraphrase some of the views, from just a few of the many who have inspired me.

Temple Grandin is a legend and an inspiration for autistic people

Ken Robinson has been outspoken on creativity in education

Cherrie Florance[10] solved the mystery of her unreachable, untouchable, silent son and now tours worldwide to share her skills.

John Holt, Oliver Sacks and Thomas West have enhanced our understanding of the concept of the mind's eye

Stanislas Dehaene[11] and Sally Shaywitz[12] have explained the neuroscience of dyslexics.

Richard Branson, together with Kate Griggs, is promoting the strengths of dyslexics through his charity #madebydyslexia

Steve Silberman has explored the history of autism and Asperger's and published many articles on neurodiversity.

Martha Herbert and Mark Hyman have exposed the connections between the gut and learning differences.

Norman Doigne has explained the science behind brain plasticity that enables students to create a new learning experience.

Robert Dilts documented the NLP spelling strategy in The NLP University Press,[13] following research by Tom Malloy[14] and F. Loiselle.

Robert Mellilo, like me, has explored the connections between all learning difficulties. He focuses on the right/left brain connections from early life.

Taking a more energetic approach, Lorraine E Murray's work *Connected Kids* and *Calm Kids* offers skills for different meditation techniques,

Claire Wilson explains the importance of being grounded, and Ober, Sinatra and Zucker explain the physical details of earthing.

Carol Dweck's invaluable work on mind-sets and Howard Glasser's Nurtured Heart Approach are invaluable to help turn around disaffected children.

And where do I fit in with this revered company? When I read works like these, I find more pieces of the jigsaw puzzle, but the picture I have created is my own and seems to be unique. To help you on your journey, I present here words both from my personal and professional experiences and drawn from several others. This journey will take you through understanding mental images, how we create them, what we use them for, how best to control them for all aspects of thinking and learning, and how things can go dramatically wrong. Let me start you on your own journey; I hope you will find it answers many of the questions you may have.

Bringing Me to Today

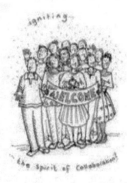

Now I'm lucky enough to be doing what I consider the best job in the world. I'm an inveterate puzzle-solver. The challenges of learning differences can be the greatest puzzles of all for an individual to unravel. Fortunately, the clues and keys lie within us.

I am now an NLP Master Practitioner, Accredited Energetic NLP Practitioner, a Thought Pattern Management Master Practitioner and a Certified Coach. These programmes have enabled me to continually refine the Empowering Learning™ processes I offer to clients. It's a great privilege to be there at the moment when people first glimpse what they can achieve.

As a Director of The International Association for Health and Learning (www.tiahl.org), which now owns all of the Empowering Learning™ materials for prosperity, we have Empowering Learning™ master trainers who instruct people around the world. Together, we coach individuals and families to understand the strengths and, in many instances, to overcome, the negative symptoms and causes of learning differences.

I have become an expert on how people learn visually and how they can make the best use of their visual skills. Creative visual learning is an exceptional skill that is currently woefully under-acknowledged.

Now, I love to read, spell quite well and have published six books, including *Seeing Spells Achieving,* which was my first book focused on improving literacy. *Bridges to Success* then took this learning further, examining other challenges. I pride myself on writing books that anyone can understand with no previous skills required.

Collaboration is always essential, and this book many contains references to other people's work. A generative collaboration, where the result is more than the individual parts, is the key to achieving this change for future generations and a vehicle for supporting further research into the areas covered in this book. To create change in any system, you need a mixture of practical experience, research, influence and motivation.

My dream is to be able to couple my ability to see different perspectives with my unabashed enthusiasm, for believing anything is possible – if we know how to do it. Using this open frame enables people to transform learning difficulties and shine.

Like my clients, I want readers of this book to say, "That makes sense"; "I feel like a kid with a new toy!" and "You seem to know my child." We all have the answers inside us, and we can benefit from some clear signposts.

Clients are almost invariably dumbfounded that no one mentions mental imagery when it is such a vital skill for all learning and so easy to master. My dream is to change this for every child.

Neurodivergent learning through the lens of mental imagery.

3.
Exceptional Strengths of EPIC Students

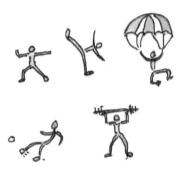

Let me remind you of my definition of EPIC students. They are exceptionally perceptive, imaginative and creative individuals. They are typically thinking and learning in neurodivergent ways, across a vast spectrum that may not match the way they are generally taught.

We have studied children and adults with exceptional strengths and explored how they do what they do well, while often challenged by learning differences. We have extended our enquiry to cover:

- Chess champions, great story-tellers, maths geniuses, those who build Lego or flat pack furniture without resorting to the instructions, those who have the most unusual ideas, etc.
- Adults who might excel in elite sports, marketing, design, garden design, business, acting, physiotherapy, etc.
- Those who rapidly recover from injury.

We believe our sample's strengths are borne out of exceptional mental imagery or something I have called "Visual Business Decisions," used by successful entrepreneurs and marketeers.

Of course, there are untold numbers of other successful people who share some of these strengths, but are not hindered by the challenges that EPIC students have to address.

To be able to maximise the use of these exceptional strengths, it is vital to shift the paradigm away from focusing on deficits to noticing strengths.

EPIC students have that something special, a unique way of looking at the world, a perspective that others often do not and cannot understand, until they meet another – it takes one to recognise one. **Misunderstood greatness.**

Several people have developed this area, using various methods, including, for example, Ken Robinson's book "The Element," Thomas G West's "Seeing What Others Cannot See," and the #madebydyslexia[15] charity.

This chapter will attempt to help you notice and appreciate the strengths of EPIC students, another **Elephant in the Classroom**. I hope it will arouse your curiosity as to how they do what they do, and discover the exceptional mental images which underpin them. Exceptional auditory skills, such as those of musicians could certainly be added, but they are not the focus of this book.

In Appendix C you will find a short form for reference.

"Visual thinking is a tremendous advantage"
Temple Grandin

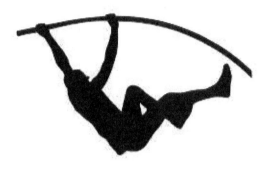

Dr Temple Grandin has designed one-third of all the livestock-handling facilities in the United States. She has autism with incredible skills to visualise the best environment for animals, so they remain calm, by putting herself into their world through her vivid imagination.

We tend to think everyone sees things in the same way we do. But wait, have you ever had the experience of going to a movie with a friend and discussing it afterwards? It can seem like you have seen two entirely different movies! "People throughout the world are on a continuum of visualisation skills ranging from next to none, to seeing vague, generalised pictures, to seeing semi-specific pictures, to seeing, as in my case, in very specific pictures," said Temple Grandin. Sometimes images can be very clear; at other times, you just "know" what something looks like, maybe the images stem from your conscious awareness. Ask yourself, "What are your mental images like?"

Ask students to describe something or someone they are familiar with. They will naturally start describing their images whether or not they are consciously aware of them. Be careful to avoid picture envy, if other peoples' pictures are better than yours. You will learn much with just a few simple questions, such as asking students to explain their favourite activities or places. With practice, they will be more consciously aware of their images, and you may be able to improve yours too.

Here are some examples of what is possible:

On YouTube there is a remarkable video of Stephen Wiltshire, the "Human Camera,"[16] reproducing all the buildings of Rome in great detail after just one trip over the city in a plane.

Elite sportsmen and women have been using visualisation skills for decades to hone their performance skills.

Boris was a pole vaulter. Pole vaulting is a very complex skill that employs excellent visualisation skills. For example, you need to be able to accurately space your run-up, carry the pole, place the end correctly in the cup, know precisely how to 'climb' the pole, launch yourself over the cross-bar and land safely. Athletes will practice this many, many times in their head during training and competition.

One of the most astounding applications for mental imagery is in recovery from a physical injury like a broken leg or operation, and anyone can do this.

When you are lying in a hospital bed in pain, getting up and moving around seem to be tough tasks. Ben had to have lots of help from the nurses or physio each time he wanted to move or get out of bed. I sat down next to his bed and asked him to visualise getting up and walking across the room. He repeated it several times until he could do it without any discomfort, as a mental exercise in his mind. A few minutes later, while taking the necessary safety precautions, he got out of bed and walked across the ward unaided!

Architects and designers can slice and dice buildings easily in their imaginations, seeing them from different angles, even converting 2D to 3D in seconds and designing new products. In short, they are picturing what others cannot see.

As another example, in *Bridges to Success* you can read about Glen, the Senior Director in an electronics company on Page 26.

Types of Mental Images

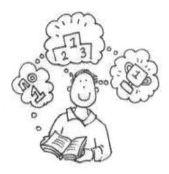

There are three types of mental images – things we have seen before and can recall, things we want to create and images that just come to us in a sort of knowing. Let me explain this in more detail.

- Things you have seen before are called **Visual Recall** or visual memory. Visual recall enables us to recognise people we know, objects, locations, events, experiences and so much more. This activity in your brain is centered in the occipital lobe. In addition, there is an area on the edge of the occipital lobe called the Word Form Area, where we hold words we have seen before, to enable us to achieve word recognition in less than 150msecs (less than a heartbeat), once we have seen the word once or twice.

- **Visual Constructs** are the things we want to create and the font of imagination. These are the pictures you dream up in your head; the things you would like to do, such as creating imaginary friends or a new dinosaur, telling stories, seeing how jigsaw puzzle pieces fit, planning the best moves in chess, picturing success in sports or just being able to learn to walk again after an injury. Note, that people with exceptional visual recall can be slightly apprehensive about visual constructs, as they don't have a ready-made picture for a new experience.

Archie had been to the same shoe shop several times and got used to the experience. When Archie's mum discovered it had closed down, she told Archie that they would need to go to a new one. Terror came across his face, and a meltdown took over. It seems that these EPIC kids have such great mental images of the past that the future without solid pictures terrifies them. She then got together some pictures of the new shop from the inside and the outside and introduced them before going on a trip.

I remember asking a young adult how she would go about redecorating her room. She then gave me the following brilliant description. I would think of the room, fade out all the furniture and the coloured walls – "so old school now," she said. Then she imagined, a swatch of carpet samples and wood flooring. She went through the possibilities and selected the perfect flooring. She did the same with the walls, choosing from an imaginary colour palette; some to be painted and one to be wallpapered. Then she rolled in the furniture and furnishings that appealed to her. She could change things around and eventually picture a perfect outcome, and she could imagine walking into the room and feeling comfortable and proud of her achievements. She did all of this as a cascade of mental images in seconds; a fabulous skill for an interior designer or window dresser.

Jimmy came to me with several challenges in school; one was that he couldn't concentrate during science lessons. I enquired about the difference between a science lesson and a maths lesson, which he adored. The usual "I dunno" was the response. I said that I knew he had good mental images and asked what he saw in a science lesson. "Oh," he said sheepishly, "I am playing on a PlayStation game in my head." "Wow that's clever," was my response. "How long does it last?" I asked. "About 20 minutes," was his reply. "Tell me, how big is the television screen you are running it on?" "That would be a 36-inch flat-screen TV," he replied with great pride. "And can you see the teacher past the TV set?" I enquired, "Not really" was his answer. In order to clarify I checked, "You are playing a PlayStation game on a huge TV set right in front of you during science lessons. And when the teacher asks you a question you haven't got a clue as to what she was talking about." "I guess" was his answer. "Do you do the same in maths lessons?" "Well, the TV is smaller, so I can hear the teacher and I do calculations at the same time. This short intervention provided many answers regarding his behaviour, and he realised that he had a conscious choice as to whether he engaged with the class.

- Finally, there are those pictures that just come to your mind. Some people call these **psychic pictures;** they are things you just know, and you don't understand why, especially when it's about someone you are close to, or "tuned in to," picking up on their thoughts. These pictures feed understanding of another person, and can be a great skill as long as they don't overwhelm a sensitive person. Students need to learn how to control them to avoid creating a feeling of being unsafe; be able to turn them off, dispose of unpleasant ones, sort excess information, filter them and stop overload. The clarity of just knowing can we such a relief, when you are quiet and tuned in your intuition. Storytelling and guided imagery encourage an individual's thoughts, urging him to make his own connections.

> Freddy knew when his mum picked him up from school whether or not she was happy. If she was stressed, she would be ungrounded and talking quickly. Freddy could pick up on his mother's mood before he even saw her. A fantastic skill, for an 8-year-old, but if mum was unhappy, he would often be unhappy too.

All of these types of pictures can be still or moving like a video, reflecting the past or imagining the future.

Creativity, Imagination and Generation of New Ideas

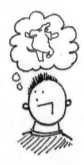

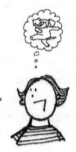

"Creativity is contagious. Pass it on"
Albert Einstein

EPIC students can have exceptional artistic talent. They may be envied by painters, artists, designers, musicians, photographers, writers and comedians. They understand pictures more than words – hence the expression "a picture is worth a thousand words." They may develop careers in the film industry, playing scenes forwards and even backwards in their imagination. They can also edit and re-run scenes before having to commit to the cutting room floor. Directors can jump into the character and know how to play the scene and then instantaneously stand back in their minds to see how the audience responds.

They may have new ideas appearing at lightning speed, sometimes too fast for others to keep up with them! Several companies now deliberately recruit EPIC employees, including Microsoft, GCHQ, NASA (see their research[17]), the armed forces and even a design house in New York that only employs those with these skills.

Fashion designers can easily imagine a dress that doesn't exist, going on to design it, working out how to construct it, and finishing the job.

Architects possess similar skills for imagining and constructing buildings, slicing and dicing in their mind's eye, to see the internal layouts and often designing whole towns.

For some their drawing skills are often in advance of their developmental age. Others get frustrated by not being able to transfer onto paper their great imagery, and won't draw.

Whilst talking with Archie he suddenly announced, when I asked him to picture a giraffe, that he could choose to see a real coloured picture, if he had encountered a real one, or a hand drawing if he had seen one in books or on the TV; a skill in itself.

In addition, he had a split screen in his memory, with one main picture, plus a row of pictures along the bottom of the screen so he could flick through them like using a mobile phone screen. (We called this skill his flip screen.)

When it came to checking how he could use this skill for misspelt words, I gave him the idea to cross out a misspelt word and put a big tick across the correct ones. Almost instantly, the correct one was large and the other incorrect spellings suddenly appeared, each with a cross on them.

Wonderful creativity and generalisations.

Many people are familiar with being able to visualise goals and get such clear images that they actualy manifest their desires. Being able to visulaise a healthy outcome can be really helpful to aiding your recovery from a health challenge.

If you notice a child laughing out of context that may well be due to him seeing mental images he finds very amusing.

Don was making progress with literacy, and he suddenly broke out into peals of laughter. His dad asked him to concentrate, but he couldn't stop laughing. I asked him what mental images he was seeing. He managed to answer in between giggles "Tennis," "doubles" and finally "there are two Alsatians playing tennis with two Cockerpoos!" By this time, we were all laughing. What a lovely creative brain Don has.

"Instagram[18]" for the Brain

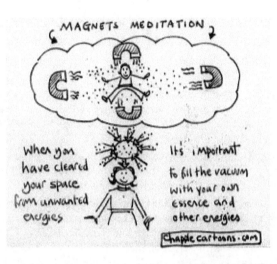

Some EPIC students have the ability to create stories from a mass of information and draw that story in cartoon form for everyone to appreciate. The translation between auditory and visual representations is invaluable for remembering any story. But this is a much more advanced skill to be able to draw together the story in real time, as someone is speaking, and present it physically on a wallchart, perhaps at a conference - the output is referred to as sketch notes. Caroline Chapple who produced many of the cartoons in this book is an expert in this area.

There has been much research into the science of drawing and memory and "there are several ways that teachers can incorporate drawing to enrich learning. Importantly, the benefits of drawing were not dependent on the students' level of artistic talent, suggesting that this strategy may work for all students, not just those who are able to draw well[19]."

Problem Solving

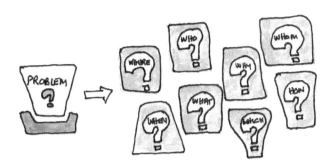

Many EPIC students thrive on solving various problems and puzzles. As you might expect, they enjoy jigsaws, chess and strategy games. They can find creative ways around most things, even their learning challenges. They create original ideas often devising really wacky ideas, thinking differently, unconventionally or seeing things from a **new perspective**; which can be summed up as "thinking outside of the box" or maybe even "failing to find the box."

Once they commit to solving an interesting problem, they can't drop it until they have found a solution – the "right" solution in their eyes. They may sometimes have to reluctantly compromise their perfectionist streaks, in the interests of completion. Insightful problem solving, can enable you to come up with a startlingly new idea, demonstrating "system-busting" skills.

> In Chapter 2 – My Corporate Career Section, you may recall my skill for solving complex problems in the medical diagnosis system. This skill is common to many IT professionals. I also find the whole area of neurodiversity something that needs better understanding – this is impossible for me to give up on.

Memory, Collecting, Concentrating and Connecting Facts

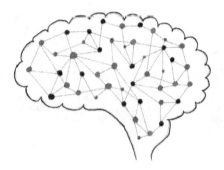

EPIC students have exceptional short and long-term memory skills and the ability to quickly perform complex mental calculations, all driven by mental images. They can exhibit incredible recall of a large amount of data such as dates, timetables, and facts and figures for anything they find interesting. Some would refer to their skills as a photographic memory. Actors can recall filming sets in great detail, knowing exactly where they needed to be to deliver lines, months and years later. Editors can hold, a whole book in their head, in order to plan restructuring. Many people have an incredible memory for football statistics, often better for matches they have watched, even recalling the goals.

They are quick thinkers, with lightening-speed abilities to make connections between different facts, noticing patterns in things that others may not see. They can gather unusual and unique insights very quickly, without going through a more traditional, slower linear process.

> The UK TV series "Death in Paradise" is a perfect example of how the detective, Humphrey, played by actor Kris Marshall, billed as being slightly dyspraxic, can suddenly resolve all the competing facts and bring together a solution to the murder, which he then explains to the suspects, how the crime was committed. You will also notice this in the Poirot series.

Hyperfocus, Drive and Energy

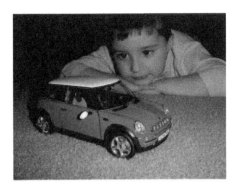

Hyperfocus enables EPIC students to exhibit a single-minded concentration on what they consider to be an interesting task or subject. Given an exciting project to work on, they are entirely absorbed, there is no stopping them! Hyperfocus can be a valuable skill in, say, the IT industry, when they are older.

EPIC students can concentrate on small details and any changes in detail. Focusing on minutiae, usually visual, can enable EPIC students to switch off peripheral vision, and block out everything else to avoid sensory overload. This is a lifesaver for those on the ASD spectrum, and a great skill for anyone working in a noisy environment.

Of course, for topics they are less interested in, EPIC students may struggle to be motivated to carry out a task they consider boring. One way around this may be to focus on the bigger question of WHY such activity is essential.

Focusing on something they really want to do provides EPIC students with more energy and commitment to the topic.

Taking Different Perspectives

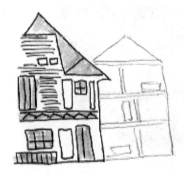 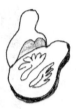

They can not only imagine what physical objects look like from different perspectives, including cross-sections, they can slice and dice buildings in their mind's eye to, for example, check internal layout, connections for utilities services, and load-bearing walls. I created the word "Perspectius", to mean genius-level ability to see different perspectives simultaneously, as it seemed an apt description for many EPIC students.

They can also picture, without any difficulty, the other side of a business opportunity or argument that others may not see. A great skill for an adult, in for example government, but it can be infuriating for families, when a child always, "takes the underdog's view."

Seeing the Bigger Picture

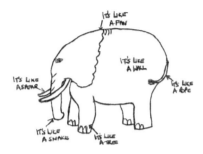

EPIC students ask "big questions," "life's larger questions," which are often challenging questions. They are curious about how things work. To aid their memory, EPIC students seem to need to have an understanding of the bigger picture, which is often accompanied by an insatiable appetite to understand the underlying reasons for every situation. They see the whole elephant in the cartoon, not just the individual parts.

They also believe that the application of creative thought best tackles problems. Rigid, ritualistic systems are considered just boring, archaic and outdated; EPIC insights fuel "system busting."

> I was working with a boy in GCSE year who loved history. I asked him what he had learnt in the last year and what made it essential. I was astonished at his understanding of the importance of history; his ability to see the bigger picture and grasp how it related to all aspects of life today with a deep understanding and an ability to explain and translate the concepts.

Visual-Spatial Thinking and Learning

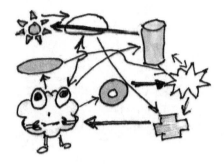

EPIC students think and learn in still pictures and/or moving videos, often possessing an extraordinary ability to recall visual memories from movies, video games or actual events. This technique is invaluable for rapid recall and particularly useful when working in the media. They need to develop the skill to switch between still and moving images, depending on how they are using the images. Attention to visual details is invaluable in all forms of media continuity.

Some EPIC students may have the ability to turn 2D images into 3D images, e.g. they can read maps, charts and graphs easily. When looking at an Ordnance Survey map, which is flat, some people can readily turn the 2D contour lines into 3D images of mountains and hills in their mind's eye.

As an example, you can read in *Bridges to Success* about David on page 25, who was a dyslexic trainee mountain guide.

Exceptional Interpersonal Skills.

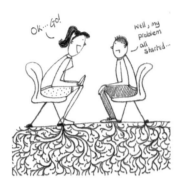

EPIC students can create verbal communications with a rich and interesting advanced vocabulary; many have developed these skills to compensate for their lack of ability with written communication. They can have tremendous powers to connect with other people and when talking will very often be getting their triggers from mental images.

Most EPIC students may have a great sense of humour; many love to laugh and may have a knack for making others laugh, too; hopefully, people are laughing with them, not at them.

Many EPIC students demonstrate strong opinions/feelings, with clarity and obvious authenticity. They exhibit a compulsion to be authentic, exhibit ethical values and express their true selves which others may find difficult to hear. See quote from Greta Thunberg about Asperger's[20]; however, they are fond of telling you exactly how it is. They see things as they really are and have a strong instinct to question and dismiss information that conflicts with their instincts. Searching out the rationale behind an instruction, helps them verify that it has an authentic purpose, or they will work to change it.

Many EPIC students bond strongly with plants and animals, enjoying the peaceful nature, as long as their anxiety is not triggered.

Intuition

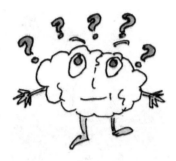

EPIC students are typically highly sensitive and warm-hearted. They can see inside people and tend to share their suffering. They often have an advanced ability to empathise. However, they usually have enough problems dealing with their own emotions, without picking up other people's feelings. To guard against picking up other people's stuff and drowning in sensory overload, they may naturally close down compassion, intuition, empathy, peripheral vision, seeing different perspectives and much of the outside world. Without these deletion skills, they will enter fight, flight, freeze or shutdown.

They can guide themselves by just knowing, often without understanding, exactly how or why they know and are frequently guided by imagery to rapidly connect disparate facts. They can see through any façade to the essence of things and people. Physical body workers and healers are perfect examples of people who just know where the problem lies and how to resolve it.

It is worth looking at popular TV, such as *The Good Doctor*, to give you some idea as to how these rapid intuitive connections lead to unique solutions, with absolute clarity as to the way forward.

Gifted and Talented

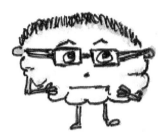

Many EPIC students have above average intelligence and may seem to be a lot older than their years. They know facts that astound you, and often have an old head on young shoulders. Many refer to this group as twice exceptional (2E), exceptional gifts and exceptional learning difficulties. There is much research appearing around this topic that intersects with EPIC students.

There seems to be a strong relationship between neurodivergency, and gifted and talented. To sum up the situation for me, it looks as if gifted children may not be identified because too often their unusual behaviours are wrongly attributed to a learning disability. Gifted and talented students have lots of neurodivergent skills, and Hans Asperger referred to his students as "little professors." From the viewpoint of mental imagery, Asperger's can look similar to gifted and talented, once mental images are brought under control. You may also come across the terms savant abilities[21] and indigo children[22].

I see synesthetic abilities, also found in some savants, as being exceptional skills. "It's a trait, like having blue eyes, nothing is wrong, synesthetics have superior memories," and "we are all synesthetics at some level." The cross-linking of senses is typical of synaesthesia which comes from Syn (together) with aesthesis (sensation), when people associate colours with letters, numbers and emotions such as pain. They can also taste words (e.g. the word cat creates a taste of peanut butter). There are thousands of examples like this on this website[23] and others offer useful examples. Research work on synaesthesia may provide an example of how abnormal network connections can form in the brain and inform research into autism, ADD etc.

The first student I met who had been identified as gifted and talented, bowled me over with his skills for using mental imagery; this was undoubtedly the source of his exceptional skills.

He wanted to tell you his own story: "My name is Ben, and I'm eight years old. I found out I was dyslexic one year ago when I was 7 and a half. I went for the dyslexia test because I wasn't good at reading or spelling or handwriting. I felt a bit confused at school, and like I was missing out on some lessons. I also felt slow and not clever when we had to read at school.

"After I found out I was dyslexic my mum took me to meet Olive. She taught me how to visualise words by taking pictures with my mind. The first word she taught me was 'train'; she wrote it on a Post-it note, and I had to imagine a picture of a train and put a picture of the word on it. Once I had a picture in my mind of the word, I could read the letters to spell the word, I could even read them backwards. It sounds a bit complicated, but I found it easy to do. Then I practised at home with ten words a day. Olive told us to use words from something I was interested in, so I chose Harry Potter. I felt very proud of myself when I could spell Dumbledore and Voldemort forwards and backwards!

"Since seeing Olive, I feel much more confident at reading and spelling at school. I usually get full marks on spelling tests and learning my spellings is very quick and easy. It only takes me about 5 seconds to visualise a word. I read much faster now, and I enjoy it more.

"It was good that I found out I was dyslexic and went to see Olive because I now feel happier, much smarter and more confident at school."

Ben has exceptional mental imagery skills, and I am delighted he found out how to use them so quickly for literacy. It's a pity he wasn't taught when he was much younger. It would have avoided any feeling of not being smart for this highly intelligent young boy.

Visual Business Skills

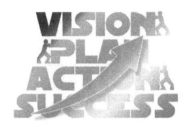

Many entrepreneurs may not think they have strong visual skills, but when you talk with them, they have, what I call "Visual Business Skills." They can imagine a new business, envision the bigger picture, see how it fits in with competitors, know the cost, estimate the volumes and calculate the profitability of any new product. This is all calculated in a flash in their mind's eye as they combine all the components. They can also have the ability to create processes and see how to step through them in the shortest time, fashioning a roadmap in their mind and then transferring it to media for others to follow. They can perform complex mental calculations quickly.

EPIC students have come up with brilliant business ideas even at a young age. Recently, there have been more and more businesses growing up, especially in the IT sector, founded by young minds. Creativity leads to many businesses being founded on a completely different business model, different from what has gone before, such as Uber and Airbnb.

EPIC role models

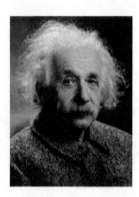

Many famous people are known to exhibit one or more of these EPIC strengths and weaknesses coupled with above average intelligence. Most of the crucial inventions and achievements in the last 100 years have been made by people who struggled in school, showed many neurodivergent strengths and become world renowned later for their accomplishments. A key is that they remained resilient and dedicated to their chosen field.

Here are just a few of my favourite examples. I invite you to pick your role models from celebrities and people you know. As I have said before, they can find the easy things in primary school hard, while the hard things in advanced work later in life are a lot easier.

Albert Einstein was a German theoretical physicist and author. He is one of the most influential scientists and intellectuals of all time. Einstein published more than 300 scientific and more than 150 non-scientific works and has received several honorary doctorate degrees from numerous American and European colleges. His name "Einstein" has, in the modern day, become synonymous with the word 'genius'.

Michael Faraday, the 19th-century physicist, was able to visualise non-visible electromagnetic "lines of force" as clearly as we see rubber bands.

Richard Branson, the founder of the Virgin Group, is one of the most well-known entrepreneurs of his time, as reflected in his visual business acumen and ability to picture success.

Erin Brockovich is the president of Brockovich Research and Consulting. She was instrumental as the lead investigator in constructing the case against the Pacific Gas and Electric Company in California. Her single-minded determination reflects many of the skills documented here for EPIC strengths.

Steve Jobs is best known as the co-founder and CEO of Apple. He is listed as holding more than 230 patents or patent applications related to technologies. Apple has changed an incredible number of paradigms regarding computing and portable devices.

Jamie Oliver is one of the world's most famous chefs and entrepreneurs. He once confirmed to me that it was easy for him to picture every dish in his mind's eye.

Ingvar Kamprad was the man who created IKEA. There are several lovely live mindmaps about how his dyslexia helped to create IKEA.

Some people, of course, have developed their own EPIC skills but have not become as well-known as these individuals. By telling us their stories, many have helped us create this chapter and contributed to the rest of this book. They have succeeded despite their learning differences and present with above average intelligence.

We have found many EPIC students overcome challenges experienced within a conventional learning environment, by developing a high level of resilience that allows them to focus on their strengths and thus excel.

In *Bridges to Success*, on page 26, there is the story of Glen, one of the unsung heroes.

Typically, these celebrities are the lucky ones, and it grieves me to say that not all show such resilience. I have given these examples because I am deeply troubled by those students who don't go on to succeed after struggling through childhood. They live their lives thinking they are stupid, failing to understand why they can't learn as others do. The answer is that they are thinking and learning differently and find things are difficult in school. Nobody has ever offered these students the opportunity to learn visually, by accurately employing their exceptional mental images. We can suffer from **"misunderstood greatness"** if nobody acknowledges our strengths.

As standardisation and testing become ever more critical in the education system, it is difficult for young students to develop the resilience to survive the tide of negativity they encounter if they cannot learn the way others do.

The following chapters will help you to understand and nurture EPIC students who have no idea about their strengths.

4.

Teachers Teach, Learners Learn

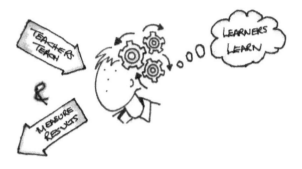

It is essential for students to understand how they do what they do – their metacognition. As the British Dyslexia Association identified in its Neurodivergent Train-the-Trainer programme, "Metacognition is one of the most impactful and cost-effective interventions."[24]

Conscious awareness of your own learning experience will assist in teaching others, so, I invite you to explore the contents of this chapter for your students and even more importantly for yourself.

Even if you have come to this later in life, Norman Doidge's work on brain plasticity highlights the human brain's ability for lifelong learning. There is no need ever to give up.

How do Students Learn?

**Phase One –
Teaching/Instruction**

Multi-sensory teaching.
Delivery of content by
teachers, tutors, and/or
parents.

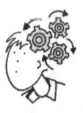

**Phase Two –
Neurological/Learning**

Processing, ordering,
storing and retrieving
information.

A fundamental part of a student's learning experience is to understand how he learns. At about six weeks old, children have learned to recognise their parents, proving they have already developed mental images. Parents will know that wearing a funny hat or a wig may cause a very young child to be confused and cry – so why does a child do that? Quite simply a child does not recognise his parents. This happens because Mum or Dad look different from the image the child has stored in his head. The mental images children form from this age have a remarkable effect on their ability to learn, e.g. recognising their toys and friends, finding something they have lost, knowing how to find their way home and so many others. All these skills use mental imagery, and everyone can do them, without these skills humans would be quite literally lost.

Phase 1 (on the left above), is the teaching stage, where teachers have been taught to teach using all of the student's primary senses; **visual** (pictures), **auditory** (sounds), **kinaesthetic** (feelings and self-talk), **olfactory** (smell) and **gustatory** (taste). These are shortened to VAKOG. Almost every learning experience includes one or more of these, and success is normally measured through results and subsequent behaviours.

In Phase 2, learners have to translate what they are being taught into an internal representation. For example, if they are read a story, they can create pictures in their mind's eye to aid their memory. But the teachers don't know what picture the student is creating unless they ask. The student is describing his or her own mental images, which may not be the same as their teacher's.

Since the Rose report about UK education, in 2009, multi-sensory teaching and learning have become accepted norms, and it is worth exploring precisely what that means. Teachers are expert in teaching; presenting information in auditory, visual, kinaesthetic and even olfactory and gustatory formats to give the student a variety of experiences.

When using visual aids in the classroom, this is *visual teaching*. However, this is only part of the first phase of the learning process and can only be evaluated, through subsequent behaviours that are not an objective measure.

The second phase of learning is the neurological phase; how information is processed and stored for retrieval. Very few teaching methodologies take into account this neurological phase. *Visual learning* is the term that should be used for the internal processing of information employing our internal visual system. This has been continuously overlooked and confused with visual teaching, possibly because it can be proven in scientific neuroscience experiments but has yet to be translated into teaching practice which requires external measurements and accurate observations. However, mental imagery is the fastest processing system. Most people use it every day, and sports coaches and athletes has been using it extensively for decades.

The quality of mental images that students create in their minds is crucial, and unless you ask the students, you have no idea what is happening in their internal worlds. Those with learning challenges can have VERY different experiences.

Let me suggest some moments of reflection about your own experiences.

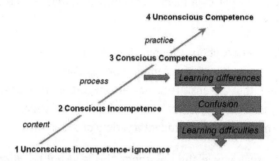

Learning New Skills

To go a little deeper, understanding the basics of the conscious and unconscious mind will also help you to know how students learn. To keep things simple, you can think of the conscious mind as containing all the thoughts the student is aware of. The conscious mind is aware only of the tip of the iceberg – perhaps 5%. There is much more under the water in the unconscious mind (95%) which is much less obvious.

As a student learns any new skill or ability, it starts as a very conscious activity. Over time and repetition, it transfers to an unconscious habit. Human beings learning new skills, pass through the four learning stages outlined below:[25]

Stage 1: Unconscious Incompetence: A state of ignorance. Not only does the student not know how to do something; he also doesn't know what he doesn't know.

Stage 2: Conscious Incompetence: Students know that they don't know how to do something. They need to learn the all-important **how to** skill: the capability.

Stage 3: Conscious Competence: They know how to do something and they need practise to become proficient.

Stage 4: Unconscious Competence: They can do something skilfully, without needing to pay attention consciously. It has become a habit.

As you are reading this, you will no doubt agree that you are breathing, but only a few people have been taught that how they breathe affects them. For example, you can learn how to breathe in a way that reduces anxiety. Similar to breathing, almost everyone is creating mental images while having little idea about how they are using them and the effects they have on their mind, body and spirit.

To illustrate this process, consider the example of learning to drive. When we are born, we are in **Stage 1**, with no idea there is such a skill to learn. At the time of your first driving lesson, you have arrived at **Stage 2**, wherein everything seems very complicated and confusing. At this stage, there are several skills to learn and a great deal of coordination is needed between looking at the road, starting the engine and braking. When you take a driving test, you are (hopefully!) at **Stage 3,** and you know exactly what to do in any given situation. After a few years of driving the whole thing has become much more automatic, and you no longer need to concentrate on the details. At this point, your driving abilities have reached **Stage 4**.

Think for a moment about how you have learned and become competent in some of your habits.

The process works in the same manner for children's education in school. In its most successful form, some youngsters may learn things in the classroom so quickly that they jump from Stage 1 to Stage 4, without apparently passing through any of the intervening stages. Others may get stuck between stage 2 and 3; they are just not learning in the same way as their peers. They then get confused, so do their parents and their teachers. They say "Nobody understands me." Why, with all this effort, is it just not working? The result is a diagnosis of learning difficulties. Fair enough, they are having difficulties in learning, but there is more than one way to learn, as borne out by the highly successful famous people mentioned earlier.

Sensory Input and Sensory Overload

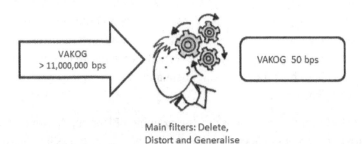

Main filters: Delete,
Distort and Generalise

Students are continually taking in information, primarily visual, through their five senses (VAKOG), at an average rate of about 11 million bits of data per second (bps)[26].

The student's experience is primarily determined by how they filter information inside their heads. The first filters are their sensory organs: eyes, ears, etc. which you could say prevent them from taking in everything around them. Their previous experiences determine the next level of filtering; memories, the language used, understanding of words and gestures, making decisions, selecting patterns in information, their values and beliefs, plus their overall attitude. They delete, distort and generalise information, hopefully discarding 99.9993% of it, thus typically reducing the information from 11Mbps to just 50bps, which is not only exceptional filtering but also quite reasonable for most people. Their internal world, behind the filters, is where the learning happens in their internal VAKOG senses, triggering a memory, emotional states and psychological responses. Currently, the results are purely measured by behaviour, but that is only a small part of the experience.

Sensory overload happens when the information in their internal conscious world exceeds the typical 50bps, with the student, experiencing an overwhelming desire to "'get me out of here." Students in sensory overload typically have their eyes flashing around, become confused and oversensitive to touch and noise, are ungrounded, may feel "wired," will over-react, fidget or just "zone out." One or more of the following can cause this:

- Excessive external stimuli, such as going into a noisy shopping precinct.
- Reduction in filtering, usually as a result of being nervous, anxious and hence very ungrounded.
- Having a VERY fast brain that creates information faster than it can be processed.
- Multiple messages from internal organs that are signalling some form of distress, for example, stomach discomfort.

People, therefore, experience any given situation differently. Their internal representations (subjective perceptions) determine how they view the world and everything they experience. For example, take five people and show them a red snake, their reactions will be different, conditioned by previous experiences of the colour red, snakes, slippery animals, etc.

Some people can wake up in the middle of the night when everything externally is quiet but their brain is racing through a "to do" list or some creative project so fast they are in sensory overload. In fact, sensory overload is very good at keeping you awake.

Some EPIC students may have pictures flying around so fast they can't keep them still. This "difficulty" is a fabulous creative skill for making up stories, animation, marketing or graphic design, but having moving letters would be a poor strategy for remembering how to spell words. In such cases, students need an additional skill to help them regain control of their visual memory, and allow them to focus on still pictures. Unfortunately, if no one notices a young person using the wrong strategy, it can result in mounting confusion.

Again, think back: When have you had moments of sensory overload and how did that experience make you feel?

Uncovering Internal Experiences

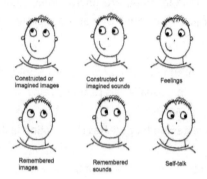

| Constructed or imagined images | Constructed or imagined sounds | Feelings |
| Remembered images | Remembered sounds | Self-talk |

So, if all this is going on inside someone's head, how do you find out what his experience really is? You can learn something by watching his eye movements as these movements generally reflect how he is accessing his internal world. Most students naturally:

- Look up for visual (V); for example, to access remembered mental images of previous experiences or making up pictures of things they want to do.
- Look sideways for auditory (A); for example, recalling a favourite tune or composing a new one.
- Look down for kinaesthetic feelings (K) and self-talk; when someone is unhappy or listening to a negative internal voice, for example, he is nearly always looking down.

Many EPIC students have exceptional mental images, and you will notice how often they are looking up. That is when they are accessing their mental images either consciously or outside of conscious awareness. People may not even be aware of these movements or even their internal images, because they happen so fast. In addition, the emphasis on looking to the right or the left is sometimes reversed, there is nothing wrong; this is just how someone is, like being left- or right-handed.

So, why is this important when teaching EPIC students? The more students understand, in sufficient detail, how they are processing information and their own experiences of learning, the more effective they will then be.

One golden rule is: "Don't let the student look down until his confidence grows." Looking up will help to avoid negative emotions and dismiss that internal gremlin who might be saying "I am stupid." As his confidence grows, the gremlin will change to "I can do this."

We have observed that our senses are somewhat like a mixing desk. Most people's senses all play their part at an even "volume." Just recall a good event in your life, what do you remember? The image, sound, feeling, taste or smell; you may have a bit of each or perhaps one is more dominant.

EPIC students and those in deep stress, tend to be more extreme, for example:

- They may look up when they are talking to access mental images and often to avoid eye contact.
- They can often be overwhelmed with too much visual information and zone out.
- Auditory can be very low or extremely loud. Autistic students may run around with their fingers in their ears, to try to reduce the volume.
- Kinaesthetic may be non-existent or overwhelming to the point of melt-down with too many negative emotions.
- Self-talk is frequently very negative, holding students stuck in "I can't."
- When talking with people about their specialist visual subject, on which they are very confident, their auditory communication may improve.

Many people think they are kinaesthetic learners, but most often they are actually visual learners, too. For example, if you learn by doing, things – like carpentry – you are using both kinaesthetic and visual skills.

EPIC students are often very short of positive internal dialogue. These students are so up in the clouds and ungrounded, they are super V (a bit like Superman), poor A and non-existent K and internal dialogue. This means they are awful at emotions and a disaster when it comes to common sense, such as crossing the road, performing random actions, making thoughtless comments, having no conscience, and they may even appear deaf when ungrounded and stressed. In addition, taste and smell are often very sensitive.

These levels are NOT fixed; they may change instantaneously, depending on the circumstances.

I met a lady in Holland, who had several challenges that made her very ungrounded. Once she was grounded, which took a little practice, she looked quite shocked, saying, "I have never felt like this before." After she took out her hearing aids, she said, "Now, I can hear." Not being grounded affects many bodily functions including hearing, you may have the volume right down or much too high.

Metacognition - How Do They Do What They Do?

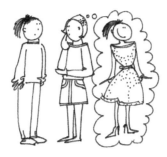

Now that you have explored the external cues; people always ask me how I know how they are using mental images. My simple answer is you **ask them!** Get them to talk about something they are enthusiastic about or familiar with. Unobtrusively, watch their eyes and notice any hand movements and you will soon have a very clear understanding of how they do what they do. You will also notice that people often don't value their strengths; they think everyone can do what they do. For example:

- The chess champion clearly saw the chess pieces in his mind's eye and could go forward several moves to see how he and his opponent would move.
- An interior designer described in great detail a house she was working on and the planned contents of every room.
- A shop window designer visualised every window, in great detail, before drafting the design for others to review.
- An actor from one of the popular soaps recalled the set he was currently working on in minute detail, including the places he needed to stand. It was an extraordinary description to listen to. He then went on to say that he could remember every set he had ever worked on.

Having discovered their underlying visual strengths, you and the student can plan how to use them elsewhere, but first, I need to explore motivation.

A Growth Mindset

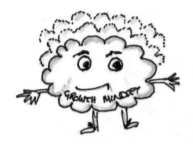 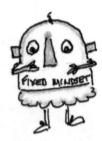

Making changes can be taxing. Critical to any learning experience is a motivation; to have a goal the student wants to achieve and, more importantly, to believe he can achieve. It also needs to be the student's goal, not just his parents'. Many of our EPIC students present being completely demotivated, believing they can't do what is being asked of them in literacy, numeracy, concentration, behaviour and paying attention. In short, all aspects of academic work. The "I can't do it" or "I'm stupid" expressions become all too familiar.

The work of Carol Dweck in *Mindsets,* identifying fixed and growth mindsets, is invaluable here, helping students see how to develop these new skills that help them progress towards their goals. Henry Ford's quote "Whether you think you can or you think you can't — you're right," is very appropriate. Most people like to be right. A **fixed mindset** believes that intelligence is static, although Norman Doigne's work on brain plasticity confirms just the opposite, supporting lifelong learning. A fixed mindset leads to a desire to look smart, therefore those who exhibit such a mindset tend to avoid challenges, become defensive, give up easily, see any effort as fruitless or worse, ignore useful feedback and feel threatened by the success of others. A **growth mindset** sees that intelligence is developed, leading to a desire to learn and therefore a tendency to embrace challenges, persist in the face of setbacks, see the effort as the path to mastery, learn from criticism and find lessons and inspiration in the success of others.

Take a moment to reflect on your own mindset and whether you believe, that with practice, you can see yourself helping others. And what is your mindset when you meet a new student, do you think they will be able to achieve improvements that are the keys to success. For me, I believe students can achieve anything they want; I just need to work with them to find out how.

Working with elite athletes recently, I found individuals very open to change because in their sport they are used to trying things to get incremental improvements – a perfect example of growth mindsets. When you praise someone be very careful to make it descriptive of exactly what you have observed. So instead of saying you "are great", which they may miss if that is not how they think about themselves, say something like, "That picture is lovely, the colours go so well together." So, you are making your praise very specific and preferably visual to match their learning style.

The Effects of Stress on Memory

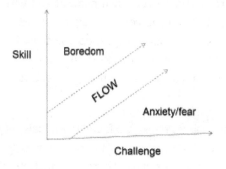

Any everyday activity can easily create stress. Stress adversely affects memory[27]. Some students may even be born with elevated levels of stress they have picked up from their mother during pregnancy or early life; many more generate it during their first learning experiences.

This diagram[28] above shows how important it is to get the balance right between the number of challenges presented to students regarding the level of skill they have. If the skill is greater than the challenge, boredom will set in, and if the challenge is greater than the skill, anxiety and fear will emerge. Empowering Learning™ processes aim to help students to get into their "flow," one step at a time.

So, whether you are working with a student in class or at home, getting into a state of being relaxed and alert is essential. Both you and the student need to practice this, for stress is contagious and extremely detrimental to creating and retaining mental images.

Use of the Occipital Lobe and the Word Form Area

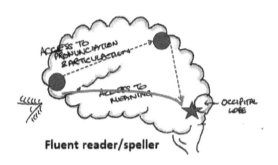

Fluent reader/speller

When children are born, they have very few mental images, and by six weeks old children can normally recognise their parents, proving that they have already developed mental images.

Around the age of 2, children have typically managed to grasp the meaning of words and shortly afterwards how to pronounce them. So, these areas of the brain have already learned some fundamentals for literacy. In addition, neuroscience has told us that the occipital lobe stores more and more pictures as students grow up which can be roughly categorised as faces, objects, locations and no doubt many more visual topics that are unique to the individual such as sports techniques and favourite holidays. The occipital lobe, is in the back of your head, just above the dent at the top of your neck – maybe this is where the expression "having eyes in the back of your head" came from! So, when you access an image of your dog, cat or family member these images come from your occipital lobe, for recognition.

Adjacent to the occipital lobe is the Word Form Area, or as Stanislas Dehaene prefers to call it "The Brain's Letterbox." The Word Form Area plays a significant role for someone who is successful at literacy, connecting the occipital lobe to the areas for pronunciation, articulation and meaning, creating people who are fluent readers and capable spellers. "Whenever subjects looked at written words, the region dedicated to vision, situated at the back of the head, was activated. Another small region of the left hemisphere, right at the border between the occipital and temporal lobes, also showed up – that he termed 'The Brain's Letterbox.'" This research has often been replicated.

Some people only use their occipital lobe for pictures, while others develop images for:

- Recalling all sorts of academic information visually.
- Developing sporting skills.
- Improving memory.
- Literacy: Spelling, fluent reading and comprehension.
- Mental arithmetic.
- Entrepreneurship.

Empowering Learning™ processes teach students how to trigger the Word Form Area and the occipital lobe for literacy and other aspects of visual learning. Teaching these skills is so quick and easy using Empowering Learning™.

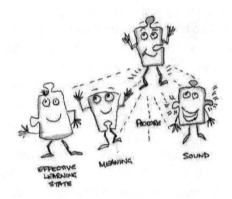

"Relentlessly Curious, Always Learning"
Leonardo Da Vinci

"I am still learning." – Michelangelo at age 87.

"Learning is the one thing the mind never exhausts, never fears and never regrets." – Leonardo Da Vinci.

Of the thousands of dyslexics, we have met, they all have one thing in common. **Dyslexics are not reliably visualising words**. Many have been resilient, got around the challenges and are successful in other ways. Others have failed and have grown up being ashamed of themselves. **Of the hundreds of EPIC students, we have met, none have discovered how best to use mental imagery for all aspects of thinking and learning.** We are always learning new skills and how these hard-to-reach people can be encouraged to find an alternative way or the most appropriate career, capitalizing on their strengths.

Several years ago, during a presentation at the University of Hertfordshire, there were several experts in special needs in the audience. I said that autistic people normally have great mental images. One lady in the audience said, "No, they don't" and her colleague, sitting next to her, said, "Yes, they do." They were both lecturers in education. Talking about this later, we all agreed that they normally have fabulous pictures of things they have seen before (known as visual recall) and often no pictures of something new they have never seen before (known as visual construct). This was a brilliant example of triggering more learning.

We encourage all Empowering Learning™ Practitioners to keep an open mind as to possibilities, hold a picture of success and to keep learning.

Alphie found remembering what he read exhausting and overwhelming. I simply asked him how he was doing it; what was his strategy. He said he made a picture in his mind for every word he could but complained that some words didn't have pictures and his brain filled up too quickly. I have never heard of anyone recommending this, so I taught him the Empowering Learning™ way of creating a picture for a sentence or paragraph as an aide-memoire. He was so pleased and said, "That's a lot better," and it also helped him avoid overload.

Feedback from parents who learn the techniques for visual learning can be embodied in the sentence: "**That makes so much sense**." They can also see the new skills helping them too.

Neurodiversity brings into focus that a considerable number of people think and learn in different ways that do not match the neurotypical way that is the focus in schools. Increasingly, people realise that these young people and adults learn differently but don't know how to ensure that the skills they are using work effectively.

Brain plasticity or neuroplasticity, as described by Norman Doigne, ensures lifelong learning. We should never give up. The brain, rather than being something static, carved out of stone that is inherited and cannot change, is more like plastic and thus malleable.

This chapter has provided information about how people learn and the processes that enable a parent or teacher to recognize clues about how their students are learning and where they might be struggling. The use of the occipital lobe and the Word Form Area is an example from the neuroscience of fluent literacy. I have covered the all-important growth mindset that sets students up for incremental success in flow and thus avoiding anxiety. Some key elements of learning differences are identified, and you will have seen how the learning process can get hijacked by confusion. Using the right strategy for your brain avoids this confusion.

In the next chapter, I will explore the inconsistencies that are apparent in the world of learning difficulties. Then take a different perspective to explain them logically, when looking at them from a perspective of mental imagery.

5.
A New Perspective: Mysteries, Contradictions and Updating the Paradigm

Mystery

Here is the paradox: There are many mysteries and other seeming contradictions we need to explore, which don't make any logical sense and all too often, are seldom noticed. The world of learning differences and neurodiversity has benefitted from recent neuroscience. Once you shine a light on what is happening behind the obvious and approach these same questions from the perspective of mental imagery, you may find the answers are straightforward. Mental Imagery provides very simple solutions to many of these mysteries and, to me, it seems as if society is looking in the wrong places.

> A teacher once insisted we "Ask the parent's permission to visualise." But, we ask students all the time, questions like "What did you do over the weekend?" The best way to recall this is through mental images of events.

The fact that people know next to nothing about their own mental images means that they are largely neglected in education today. This book offers a new perspective based on working with thousands of EPIC students who struggle with learning. I argue that mental imagery should be a vital part of education and its absence can explain many learning differences and subsequent learning difficulties, thus shining a light on how to change the prevailing perspectives.

Please read through this chapter slowly, thinking of the EPIC students you meet. Then you will be guided through a new perspective, of mental imagery for these challenges that calls for an extension to the current educational paradigm.

Civil Rights

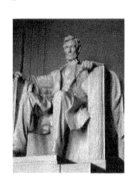

Freedom to "give everyone a fair chance in the race of life" Abraham Lincoln

We need to change the current paradigm with a new perspective to enable these students to learn in the best way for them. As Abraham Lincoln phrased it, we seek the "Freedom to give everyone a fair chance in the race of life."

Amanda Spielman, OFSTED Chief Inspector, said[29] that "children's time in education are their wonder years. A time when they get to grips with the power and flexibility of the English Language and fundamental mathematical concepts." She continued, "High-quality education, built around a rich curriculum, is a matter of social justice.... Using the definition of cognitive psychology, as a change in long-term memory, if nothing has altered in long-term memory, nothing has been learned." So, failing to assess children's visual memory, a vital part of their long-term memory, is not socially just.

Mental imagery is a vital part of learning anything, but nobody even mentions it in schools. The classroom is mainly an auditory experience, and the box for visual teaching is ticked with knowledge of visual teaching but without any knowledge of a student's visual learning. There is no teacher training in mental imagery, and it is not even mentioned in the UK's Early Years curriculum[30], contradicting the schools' commitment to multi-sensory teaching and learning. Mental imagery is a key part of visual learning – it can't be right not to teach teachers about the key role mental imagery plays in learning! Nobody ever discusses mental images and they need to be incorporated into the current paradigm. It is indeed a remarkable school with an enlightened staff that teaches students how to visualise.

By comparison, mental imagery is an accepted part of sports training, with every elite sportsperson unable to manage without this skill. For example, athletes envision the ball going into the net, the flight of a javelin and not just winning a race but having successful strategies for every part of a race. For instance, watch someone taking a conversion kick on the rugby field, or playing golf. You can see them visually following the trajectory of an imaginary ball, before making contact; you will see these skills in action. Can you imagine how a pole-vaulter, a ballerina, a high board diver or a gymnast could manage without good mental imagery for rehearsal? Elite sportsmen and women have used these skills for decades.

> Working with some athletes and mentors from the Dame Kelly Holmes Trust[31], the visual skills of all successful athletes were obvious.

This book challenges the status quo and explores something so obvious that the current paradigm is missing it. It has the potential not only to reduce the students' and their families' stress dramatically but to save the education system in many countries a fortune in special provisions. You are learning new skills based on the students' strengths, not their deficits. Referring to Thomas G West's book *Seeing What Others Cannot See*, Empowering Learning™ has quite simply seen what others cannot see, and the solution is surprisingly simple. We will consider the very definition of learning difficulties, deficits and disabilities, especially dyslexia and question whether all the effort is being put in is even addressing the right question.

Mysteries and Contradictions

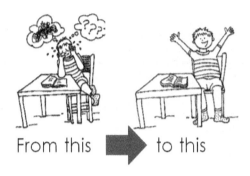

From this ➡ to this

There are several things in the education system that seem to conflict with what parents, coaches and teachers are trying to achieve with EPIC students. These become blindingly obvious when working with students in an open-frame curious way. I apologise in advance for those who already know this; sadly, there aren't that many of you.

1. Phonics may have improved reading for many, but big picture thinkers and dyslexics can't cope with the minutiae of phonics, that doesn't have any visual meaning. They find whole word recognition much more natural, which is the target for fluency in any reading strategy. Students are left to pick up word recognition by chance, whereas students could be easily checked, before they get confused, and taught in minutes.

2. Schools are committed to multi-sensory teaching and learning but, for example, 100% of the dyslexics we have met are not visualising words; 100% of those with ADHD can't control their mental images; and 100% of those we have met on the autistic spectrum are simply drowning in mental images. Teacher training does not include the vital difference between visual teaching and visual learning, which are often mistakenly thought to be the same thing and highlighted

in *"When Bright Kids Can't Learn"* by John F Heath. We are not aware of any teacher education in how students learn visually, using mental images, for all sorts of applications (spelling, reading, comprehension, remembering what you read, good handwriting, maths, memory, sport, etc.). This means that teachers and their EPIC students are being set up to fail.

3. Both the English and French languages, as well as a number of others have deep orthographic structures, meaning there is a large gap between what a word sounds like and how it is written, so students need to learn how to visualise words, to cope with homophones, silent letters, and words that break a variety of rules. Italian is considered an exemplar of a phonetic language where you write exactly what you hear, not so for English. This means for English you need mental images to read fluently and to spell.

4. For a phonic language, for example, Welsh, Italian or Spanish spelling can be very straightforward you just write what the word sounds like. Although reading is similar you still need mental imagery to progress to word recognition and fluency.

5. The students' exceptional visual strengths are not identified, nor explored, leaving what they really do well, undiscovered. Visual learning is not even mentioned in the Early Years Framework. So, it is left to chance as to how our students use their visual images. They may easily get confused by them and may even shut down.

6. Many children are stressed in school and that destroys learning. There is little focus on how to get quickly grounded, remain calm and enter into an effective learning state, which also stabilises images and words on the page. Grounding is a high-speed use of mindfulness.

7. Many dyslexics had early hearing problems (glue ear, grommets,

etc.) but are taught a purely auditory strategy with which they are bound to struggle. Even many of those with cochlear implants are taught phonetically. One boy explained that using his cochlear implant was like listening to someone while underwater and it is really difficult to hear phonemes.

8. Visual thinkers are not learning in the best way for them in a school that emphasizes primarily rote learning[32]. "They find the easy things in primary school can be hard, whilst the hard things in advanced work later in life can be easy," said Thomas G West. More advanced work requires creativity, the ability to make connections, inspiration, etc. – all the EPIC skills.

9. Reading flat on a table is unnatural, puts more unnecessary strain on struggling students, who may find letters being distorted or moving around. Looking down eliminates mental imagery and increases emotions, making matters worse. Reading with work propped up will help increase fluency.

10. Reading comics may be more comfortable as speech bubbles are typically in capitals, that don't turn around and make different letters.

11. Idioms are highly visual and are taken literally by EPIC students, who convert them to pictures and thus find they make no sense. Please try to avoid using idioms until students are coping better, with the English language.

12. Assessments are costly and time-consuming and all about deficits and failure. Where strengths are referred to, as in "no deficit" e.g. letters don't move on the page, these are not explored. More details of "how" the students do succeed, using their natural skills in, for example, cooking, art, maths, and science experiments

would assist their learning in other disciplines. This wealth of valuable information is not identified. Few reports identify mental imagery strategies for parents. In cases where they do mention such strategies, the details of the actions to be taken by schools are often inaccurate. Whilst awaiting assessment, there are many simple skills parents and children can learn.

13. Julian Elliot has explained, in the *Dyslexia Debate*, "There is no relationship between a dyslexia diagnosis and the kind of treatment, intervention and educational programme we would provide that is different or additional to that which we would provide for any adult or child struggling to read." The same strategies are offered to all.

14. Much of a dyslexia report is about assessing phonics; this is a very limited view. In addition, why bother to spell nonsense words? I know it is to test a student's phonics, but it is still nonsense and doesn't encourage word recognition. Why should students be able to spell words they have never seen before when only 46% of the words in English are spelled phonetically correct. We estimate that for every word a fluent reader wants to spell, they will have seen it before.

15. The high-frequency words, focused on in early years, have very few nouns among them to encourage the use of the occipital lobe and the word form area.

16. The whole primary maths curriculum presupposes that children visualise numbers. Mental arithmetic/maths needs mental images; the clue is in the title! People often seem to accept that it is OK to be bad at maths, thus reducing motivation to improve. Why are we learning times tables in order? They never come up in order in calculations. Some maths resources will create an overload for EPIC students, for example, addition and multiplication squares.

17. EPIC students often have above or well-above average IQs. But they are seen, and see themselves, as deficient in some way that they are unable to change.

18. People should not be ashamed of their challenges; they have just not been taught in a way that works for them.

19. There are thousands of bright, exceptionally creative people who, without using controllable mental images, find numeracy, communication, literacy and all aspects of concentration difficult.

20. We have an academic system that relies on words and numbers and neglects creative skills.

21. It is accepted that visual word recognition is needed for fluent reading, but it is neither checked nor taught explicitly.

22. Teachers, parents and support staff may have different accents which are challenging when using a purely auditory strategy.

23. The focus is typically on behaviours, and what is going on to cause these behaviours, but not the underlying problems such as literacy, numeracy, uncontrolled mental images/vivid flashbacks. There are huge gaps between mental health, behaviours and education – Sara Haboubi refers to these as "mental fitness."

24. Being highly visual can be hereditary by either nature or nurture but need not imply learning challenges.

25. Teachers in the UK have to teach phonics exclusively in reception year and year 1. However, the current SAT tests mark children down for spelling words phonetically in year 2.

26. Students who can't concentrate in class can focus on a computer for hours at home or play.

27. It is accepted that not everyone learns in the same way, and that students with the same labels have not got the same functional learning challenges. So why do we teach them all in a standardised way?

Some people have commented that the work we do is so simple, it can't possibly work. Who said a change has to be hard? Some of the best discoveries started as just a hunch. "The world is full of obvious things which nobody by any chance ever observes," says Sherlock Holmes. In our science-based world, every issue often seems to have an ever more complex solution. Perhaps this has led us to overlook the obvious!

What is invariably missed is that visual skills for learning are entirely teachable; they are not and should not be viewed as disabilities — just **Misunderstood greatness.**

Updating the Paradigm

The 7 steps to success

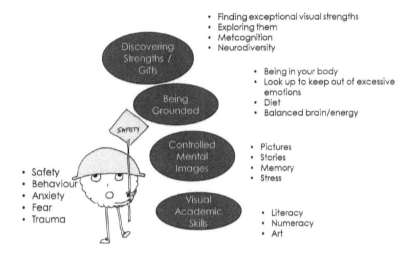

- Finding exceptional visual strengths
- Exploring them
- Metcognition
- Neurodiversity

- Being in your body
- Look up to keep out of excessive emotions
- Diet
- Balanced brain/energy

- Pictures
- Stories
- Memory
- Stress

- Literacy
- Numeracy
- Art

- Safety
- Behaviour
- Anxiety
- Fear
- Trauma

This is where all the **Elephants in the Classroom,** in this book, come together. To repair the current paradigm, the following actions are needed, for all students under age seven. Providing parents, teachers and support staff with these skills takes just a few hours, and they can teach their students in minutes. This is where the power of functional learning comes in; focusing on specific topics that the student would like to improve rather than having all the focus on which diagnoses to follow. For different challenges, you may need to focus on one area in depth, but to get started for every child, the following steps are a good place to begin:

1. Identify strengths and their metacognition to facilitate learning.

2. Reduce the students' stress and re-enforce their feelings of safety in every aspect. Teach grounding to stabilise images, release negative emotions and reduce sensory overload.

3. Teach all students how to use mental imagery for pictures, stories, memory and most importantly to keep them under control.

4. Then teach all students how to picture words for spelling, reading (in parallel with phonics for new words) and numbers (for numeracy). Focus on teaching nouns associated with pictures <u>first</u>. Leave high-frequency words until a bit later. Only progress to non-nouns on a whiteboard once you are certain nouns are secure.

5. Make this inclusive of everyone in the class, especially those with SpID and hearing impairment.

6. Monitor and improve nutrition and water intake.

7. Introduce several detailed visual tips including; propping books up for improved stability when reading, visualising number triangles for times tables, creating pictures of what you read to improve comprehension, learning how to copy down from the board without looking at what you write, improving handwriting and mind-mapping for organising thoughts, etc.

Empowering Learning™ can offer a variety of ways to learn these skills quickly and easily, including our simple study guide and CD (available at www.empoweringlearning.co.uk).

> **Child's play:** I was in a primary school one day, and the head teacher had organised all the little groups who had extra help to come with their learning support teachers to a single class. In just 45 minutes we had all the students visualising pictures and developing the skills to picture words. All went well, and they went off to their next lesson. Walking across the playground at lunchtime, I saw one of the students who had been in our class teaching one of her friends who hadn't. This technique is so simple that 6-year olds can teach it. What a delight!

Discovering Students' use of Mental Images

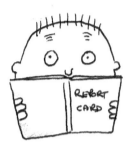

To unravel older students' confusion, you and your pupils must understand the experiences described in the following chapter, "What happens when mental imagery goes wrong." Before going there, we want to offer you, in Appendix A, some questions to help discover the students' use of mental images that could be used by parents, coaches, teachers, assessors and educational psychologists to give them more than just an auditory analysis of older students' experiences. Students and their parents need to understand the child is just missing a skill that can be easily taught, and the sooner they begin, the better.

When you take a different perspective, such as is offered in this book, change can be rapid. Seeing students succeed is a hugely rewarding experience and one that opens new possibilities, both for EPIC students and potentially for improving family life.

As you become more curious, further insights are likely to present themselves. You will become aware of other strategies for learning that will prove beneficial to you and your students. Many of my students are gifted with a genius level ability to see different perspectives simultaneously; physically, mentally or emotionally. By the end of this book, you will be able to see for yourself and those you care about, a new perspective – one that nurtures their extraordinary skills in a way that can serve them even better.

6.
When Mental Imagery Goes Wrong

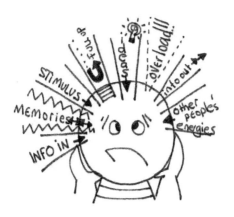

Before reading how to help EPIC students become stunningly successful, I have to flip the coin and discuss what happens when mental images, which may work well in one environment, turn out to be a nightmare in another. In short, students don't know how to get the best from their mental images, because nobody teaches them nor their teachers. Students also don't realise how to stop being overwhelmed by their own images.

This chapter is extensive because mental images can go wrong in many ways and cause a great deal of distress until you understand them. Checking them at a young age minimises all these symptoms developing. Stories are used to give more examples of our discoveries. Chapter 7 teaches students how to change their experiences if they wish.

A New Perspective - Joining the dots

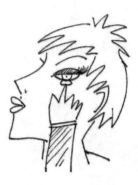

You need to consider what is behind the student's behaviour. You will need an open mind to read this chapter and start to see what is really happening for these EPIC students. This is where the golden nuggets are. I have been able to employ my skills for seeing different perspectives and explaining, through the lens of mental imagery, many of the challenges and exceptional skills. These insights are what makes Empowering Learning™ unique.

To help the reader, I have split this section into subsections, one or more of which will be relevant to specific students. Each section contains a list of symptoms. Over half of the symptoms have also been identified in the BDA's Neurodiversity Train-the-Trainer programme, under the title of various learning difficulties, without, in any way, being a diagnosis. Neurodiversity is a wide spectrum.

This chapter also identifies actions needed to improve these symptoms from the perspective of mental imagery, and points to skills to be learned in Chapter 7.

Few people are looking at how and why students do what they are doing, when they are exhibiting positive skills.

This book will demonstrate the need for extending the definition of visual learning to include what is happening inside someone's head, with their mental images – a hitherto neglected paradigm. Integrating mental imagery into teaching will benefit everyone and especially our youngest EPIC students.

When we look at applications for mental images, we find that our everyday activities are littered with them: Doing the shopping, making breakfast, choosing clothes to wear, travelling, and finding ingredients for a meal, are just a few. As far as academic work is concerned, we can, for example, recognise words, "see" how to spell them, picture them in another language, do mental arithmetic, recall mind maps, charts, images of digestion, the geography of the planet – almost anything you want to learn. It would be so helpful if students were taught how to harness these skills of mental imagery for recall and construct from a very young age. When you are very busy, there can be numerous thoughts running around in your head. This is confusing for most of us, and as adults, we learn to take a break. For EPIC students, this constant inundation is an everyday occurrence and may not be pleasant.

Mental images start with objects/faces/locations etc., when you are very young and then you progress to the need to develop for words, numbers and any other specialty area, like football or pole vaulting, as you grow up. These are really simple skills to teach and should be introduced to students who are under the age of 7. They should include pictures, words and numbers. Passing seven years old, without controlled mental images for pictures, words and numbers is going to have a significantly detrimental effect on every student's learning. Yet, it takes seconds to check and minutes to teach.

In this new paradigm, we are looking at things the other way around and striving to find the most appropriate way to reach and then teach these fantastic EPIC brains.

Limiting Beliefs sap Motivation.

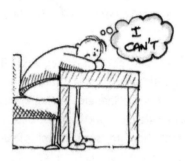

Symptoms:

- Students believe "I can't," or they may feel stupid and develop a fixed mindset, which inhibits growth and learning.
- EPIC students can be bullied for being different.
- Students feel stuck.
- There is too much focus on the relationship between familial genes.
- Assessments are generally very negative, focusing on what the student can't do.

Topics to explore:

Students can very quickly develop limiting beliefs about their abilities to read, to spell, concentrate, do comprehension, speak, etc. which may also generate limiting beliefs about themselves – "I am stupid" for example. It is often more difficult to shift a limiting belief than it is to learn a new skill, especially when you are so embarrassed about your abilities. You will find every excuse possible to avoid going back to that dark place.

A little boy, Charlie, said, "It's OK, my dad didn't learn to read until he was 45, so I have got plenty of time." I do not doubt that dad was trying to encourage his son, with the best of intentions, not to let the lad be too hard on himself, but the unfortunate outcome was that the student didn't think he needed to bother with this stuff that he found difficult. We do need to take care of how we speak to young impressionable minds.

I have met hundreds of students who think they are stupid and some who are convinced words just drop out of their heads. If we believe these things, there is no motivation to change and prove yourself wrong; we do like to be right. You need to change from a fixed mindset to a growth mindset, believing anything is possible with practice and the right supporting strategy.

Actions needed:

- When a teacher or parent believes that a student will succeed, this has a significant effect on the outcome. Unfortunately, the opposite can also be true. We must avoid these self-fulfilling prophecies. Create small steps to maximise success, and build their new visual skills on top of what they are already good at. For example, picture words on their favourite train, animal, game, whatever works for them.

- Investigate the language of creating a growth mindset. (See Carole Dweck's book *Mindsets*)

- Point out things that they are doing right, even for a few seconds, saying, for example, "Thank you, Harry, for sitting still. I can see you are really concentrating".

The Qualities of Mental Images

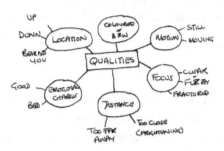

Symptoms:

- Images are too far away, difficult to see and even inaccessible.
- Images are too close and frightening.
- Students can't switch between still and moving pictures and vice versa.
- Images are fuzzy, fractured or refuse to stay still.
- Images are moving too fast to see.
- Images may not be conscious, just an awareness of what something looks like.
- Students are not looking up into their visual field to access the best mental images.
- Students are always looking down and are generating emotional charges around failure.
- Laughing out loud for no apparent reason.

Topics to explore:

The common qualities of images, known as sub modalities in NLP, are mentioned in the diagram above. In addition, you might like to add brightness, contrast, texture, detail, size, shape, border, orientation, associated/disassociated, perspective, proportions, dimensions, and singular or plural. Remember, you may be able to notice these by watching the student's eye movements. Ideal images are about 3-5 feet away, causing the student to look up to the left or right, exhibiting conscious control over movement, whether in 2D or 3D.

The qualities of EPIC students' mental images can vary dramatically from person to person, and often within one student at different times.

- Mental images too near can be terrifying, generating anxiety and fear. Just imagine a lion "in your face!!" If mental images are too far away, the student can't see them clearly, so he may seemingly drift off in an attempt to focus.
- Mental imagery moving too rapidly makes the student feel wobbly and won't work for words and numbers that need to stay still.
- EPIC students have miraculous memories of the past, but may not picture the future and hence are terrified of new experiences.

The student will find the best images by looking up and he has the choice as to where the best pictures are – to the left or the right.

Mental imagery in 3D is great for creativity but not useful for words and numbers.

Actions needed:

Chapter 7 will provide you with some tips on how to help the student get the best quality mental images as well as how to control them. Looking up is where our visual memory works best.

Not Using Mental Images

Symptoms:

- Losing things.
- Being forgetful of daily activities.
- Getting lost.
- Poor memory.
- Inability to draw.
- Finding it hard to follow more than two directions.
- May have some OCD symptoms, such as not recalling locking the front door, so going back to do it again and again.
- May have superfast images they can't see.
- Ineffective learning and problem-solving.

Topics to explore:

Sometimes students have told me they are sure that they have no mental image. There is now research being carried out into Aphantasia[33], but experiences are bound to differ between people. It may be that some just don't consciously use mental images, although they may dream in fill colour. First, you need to check out the student's expectations. Some people may see full colour, almost like a 36" colour TV, while others have black and white images. Some may have cartoon images, while others just know what something looks like, without having an actual image at all. All of these are usable. Some images move too fast for the student to retain them.

John had fantastic mental images but was always hard on his own physical pictures and threw most of them away. I asked him to compare the pictures in his head with the ones he could produce on paper. His immediate answer was, "In my head is a lot better." This is something highly visual people have to learn to live with and just practice perfecting their skills until their hand catches up. Just remember how lucky you are to have excellent images. You can always try imagining the picture on the piece of paper and use it like a stencil.

It is only a tiny percentage of people who can't recognise their nearest and dearest, so they do have pictures stored somewhere. The problem is more about how to access and use them. Of course, in extreme cases of trauma, you may have subconsciously switched them off to avoid revisiting a scary experience. I have only met two people who don't have any images at all, both of whom had brain damage. Very often EPIC students have great mental images but have not learned how to use them for academic skills.

Picture envy should be avoided when talking with others who seem to have far better pictures. The issue is generally about managing expectations and taking time out to relax and create a good mental image. Infants need mental images to recognise their parents, a vital skill for survival, and it is essential to carry on using this skill, or in Norman Doidge's words, "If you don't use it you may lose it, as other parts of the brain set up camp in that area."

Actions needed:

Chapter 7 will teach you how to start with simple topics like recalling what your cat or house looks like or part of your favourite film/TV show. As you progress, you will learn how to use mental images to improve your memory.

OCD can be improved by consciously taking pictures of actions you carry out, like locking the front door when you leave home.

Not being Grounded affects Mental Images

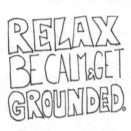
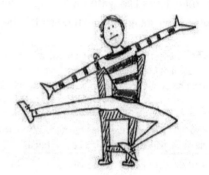

Symptoms of being ungrounded:

- Often appears clumsy, bumps into things/people.
- Has obvious good/bad days.
- Anxious and fearful.
- Poor organisation.
- Poor posture/hypermobility.
- Inconsistent performance.
- "On the go" constantly, often running around.
- Talks rapidly.
- Inability to perceive external risk/danger, such as when to cross the road.
- Can't sleep, racing mind or dreams.
- Poor balanace, struggles to ride a bicycle.
- Fidgets with hands and feet or squirms on the seat.
- Poor listening and general behaviour.

Topics to explore:

Being ungrounded, another associated **Elephant in the Classroom**, can be seen through any or several various observable symptoms listed above and the result is normally deteriorating behaviour. Mental imagery can cause people to be ungrounded, even when asleep. Relatively minor stress can create confusion and prompt students to become ungrounded. This low level of stress can be easily generated, for example, by being nervous, by trying to stretch the student outside of his skills or capabilities, or by putting him on the spot, perhaps by asking him to read aloud.

Being grounded or ungrounded is just a state that students can pop in and out of in seconds. A child can balance to ride a bicycle one minute and trip over his own feet a minute later. When students become ungrounded, we have seen examples of their natural sensory functions, "misfiring." In such a state, a student may become super visual, partially deaf, lack emotion and have no internal dialogue to warn him about risks and dangers.

You can think of being ungrounded like a sparrow in the garden; continually twitching and looking around to check whether they are in danger. Whereas the pigeon in the top of the tree is perfectly still and confident. He can focus on other topics.

Actions needed:

So, prioritise keeping students relaxed to minimise stress. Helping students to become grounded will stop their habitual stress and bring many of the symptoms under control.

Empowering Learning™ uses simple guided imagery and balanced breathing to encourage grounding. (See chapter 7.) There are some useful tools to assist the student (weighted blankets, wobble cushions[34], fish oils, coloured/tinted glasses, and sand-jackets to name a few) but I must stress that whatever you use needs to be quick as students can become instantly ungrounded mid-lesson, and from the student's point of view it is better not to be visible. You may also find that in school for example he is clumsy, but not at home when he can ride a bike; this show how being grounded and ungrounded are just transient states, depending on stress levels.

Too many Uncontrolled Mental Images

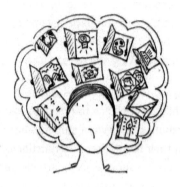

Symptoms:

- Poor concentration and focus, easily distracted and "flying off at a tangent" or "zoning out."
- Has difficulty paying attention and seems not to listen when spoken to directly.
- May develop mental health problems.
- Students are highly sensitive, reflecting others' moods intensely.
- Difficulty in organising tasks, activities or knowing where to start.
- Will have a confusing internal world with lack of organisation and chaotic internal images.
- May have their eyes flashing around frantically trying to keep up with their imagery.
- Images get knocked off the channel and seem like interference on a TV.
- Slow or struggles to respond when given instruction or asked a question.
- Multiple simultaneous video screens – distraction abounds.
- Can't cope with generic words.
- Not understanding jokes and idioms.
- Racing thoughts can feel like your brain in on fire.

Topics to explore:

These are the typical symptoms associated with ADHD and Autism; where the student received a cacophony of intrusive thoughts, visual and auditory, all at the same time, competing for his attention, with nobody is in charge. This experience is exhausting and even trying to focus on just one thing, that he is really interested in, puts extreme pressure on him. The expression a wandering mind[35] is very apt for ADHD, when a series of images connect to each other at terrific speed. Sometimes this experience can be outside of conscious awareness, so the students knows that there are hundreds of thoughts going on, but doesn't even know what they are. David Mitchell has a great summary "when you loose your ability to communicate, the editor-in-residence who orders your thoughts walks out at no notice."[36]

I often ask students to start by picturing a cat or a dog, checking they aren't frightened of either. One day I goofed up and forgot to check before I asked Amy to picture a cat. She gripped the arms of the chair so tightly her knuckles went white, and she looked terrified. I asked her what was happening. She said she had a video of 100 cats on a single screen and they were all fighting! So, I started asking her what she could do. Did some of them need food? Could she let some out into the garden, etc. until she calmed down and just had one sitting on a lovely velvet cushion? She was now in control and could make progress. Can you imagine what her experience would have been like in school if someone had mentioned cats? Thank goodness, I didn't ask her to picture a lion!!

This is where it is imperative students have balance. Multiple mental images are great for creativity, etc, as discussed in Chapter 3, but there comes a point where mental images can be overwhelming. Who can say how many are too many, but at some level the student will know what is comfortable? With too much stress, the student's sympathetic nervous system will trigger the "fight" response where behaviour can deteriorate. This level of stress can do all sorts of interesting things to mental images. Bringing images under control through grounding and mindfulness will enable the student to:

- Slow down very fast movies, which the student can find terrifying.
- Calm down and reduce fidgeting.
- Repair images that get fractured as if they were painted on a pane of glass that has been broken.
- Stop images from being "knocked off the channel" where they had appeared like fuzzy black and white dots, similar to those that you see when you turn on a TV.

> Having been asked to picture a cat, little Freddy started waving his arms across the top of his head as if he were trying to clear some cloud. I asked him what he was doing, and he said he didn't know but there were lots of spots up there, like the black and white spots you see when you first switch the TV on and he was trying to brush them away. I guessed that his pictures were moving so fast they were just a spotty blur. Can you imagine what this would be like? No wonder he was so ungrounded. After much grounding practice, he got the real pictures to appear.

With all this imagery in full flow, it is not surprising that EPIC students have difficulty maintaining attention, organising tasks, and assembling their thoughts.

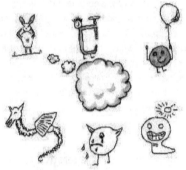

Many EPIC students have multiple mental images. These can all be on one screen or appear to the student on multiple screens, similar to a TV store where they have banks of televisions, all on different channels. When very young children experience this, it can be a source of excessive stress that can sometimes manifest itself into head-banging or other painful outlets. In conjunction with this, some EPIC students become somewhat OCD about having to watch every screen simultaneously – exhausting. You will see this in their eyes, flashing from one picture to another.

> Working with a premier league football manager, I noticed his eyes flashing continuously. I asked him how many images he was seeing. After a few moments'

thought he could explain 2-3 images that were coming into his head. I asked him what the maximum number was. To my astonishment, he said about 100 (he holds my world record), and I had no idea how he was achieving this. So, I enquired whether they were the same or different. He replied, "Well, before or while I am watching the team play, I have different strategies running on each screen and I watch each one to see how it will work out." This is an astounding skill but little did he realise that it is unlikely any team member will have the same ability. He then went away to rethink his team talks, to maximise his communication with the players. Teaching him to switch off screens, allowed him to reduce and expand his focus as he wished.

It is well known that students on the autistic spectrum struggle with generic words; for instance, teachers are advised not to use words like shoes and instead be very specific, saying for example "those blue shoes." You may think of this as a lack of ability but we 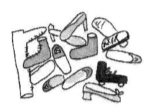 prefer to think mentioning a generic word like "shoes" creates a deluge of mental images to choose from of all sorts of different shoes, colours and sizes, with no structure at all, which puts the person into instant sensory overload.

The film about Temple Grandin, Thinking in Pictures, has excellent graphics to demonstrate this, with quite literally dozens of shoes firing towards her at the very mention of the word shoes.

Once you understand more about your own mental images, they can become your friends; a real benefit to you, in all aspects of your life. However, having no control over your mental images can be a terrifying experience, generating fear, panic, chaos, overload, lack of concentration, and being ungrounded.

People have unique "maps of the world". Please remember, one person's chaos may be another person's normal, and they may well not want to change. Tell them you have a choice. You do not need to remain stuck; it is just your current "map of the world"; all maps are changeable – a great deal of neuroscience research supports this.

> I have met so many examples - Billy who watched four different TVs in his mind every time he sat in a maths lesson and complained he couldn't concentrate. Incredible skills but at the same time overwhelming. Archie has loads of ideas; he is the most creative kid in the class, but he has difficulty communicating them. When he tries really hard, his head spins, he feels sick, he can't sit still, and he feels "all over the place." This can lead to really black moods, embarrassment, frustration, meltdowns and anger at himself.

Many EPIC students have very fast brains and hence very fast-moving pictures. They can often be stuck in movies and not able to create any still pictures. For literacy, this will cause letters and whole words to transpose, letters may fly around, disappear, run in wiggly lines and generally misbehave. This may be described as an ADHD trait, but you just need to learn how to gain control. Again, these skills are great for creativity of any kind but not for academic performance.

> M, an adult, came to me because her "brain was racing." As she described it, she kept getting distracted when speaking which isn't good when you are trying to concentrate or sleep. So, I enquired whether there was ever a time when it was calm. "Yes, golf," was her immediate reply. M had taken up golf recently, and she described all the things she had to remember for golf and how focused she was. She even gave me a demonstration, and I noticed how grounded she was. Getting her to anchor that state, especially the grounding, meant she could take that into the rest of her life. She had an obsession with never turning her iPhone off and when she was explaining anything, she would often get side-tracked, mid-sentence, to show me an iPhone picture about something related. This could even happen when she was trying to get to sleep, and the only conversation she was having was with herself. Shutting the cover of an iPhone isn't sufficient to protect yourself from the signals that may keep your brain active.

> When Mary came to see me, she was five years old and diagnosed with "slow processing." I asked her the same question that was cited in her report. "Why do you go to an airport?" I waited for about 20 seconds before she answered: "To go

on holiday in another country." "Thank you," I replied and then asked her what she was doing in the gap between me asking and her answering. She lived in Luton and explained that the car went under the tunnel and then parked in the middle between 2 other cars. Then they all got their luggage, and they saw three planes all with different coloured paint that she described. She took her pull-along suitcase right up to the terminal and then left it at the luggage check-in. Then they went up the escalator, bought a juice and a snack............and finally, she said: "To go on holiday in a different country." This child wasn't slow; she was very busy, she had perfect recall of the whole visit and just needed to re-run her experience before she came to the end result!

Those who seem to be slow and struggling to respond when given instructions or asked a question are often not slow but very busy with sorting out their pictures.

Speaking to a Taekwondo coach and Commonwealth Medallist one day, I asked him about the mental images he saw during a fight (which I always think as of chess for your feet). Sure enough, he could see his next move, then his opponent's, then his etc. Most of his images were continually moving, which is a great skill for Taekwondo. I asked him whether he ever saw any unwanted pictures. He looked at me very sheepishly and said, "Yes, when I approach the mat, I sometimes get things like how am I going to get home or what's for tea." I enquired with a smile whether that was helpful and taught him to turn off the ones he didn't need. In an instant, I taught him grounding by using the analogy to other sports, say golf and then suggested he could imagine a remote control for his extra screens and turn them off. This 6'6" Taekwondo expert looked at me and said, "The world has suddenly calmed down; thank you so much, I will go and teach my students now." One of the great things about working with athletes is their openness to new ideas. If they make a positive difference, they will embrace and develop them further for their specific requirements.

Once the student is consciously aware of all this activity and can explain it, he will start to have a choice.

Actions needed:

- Learn to control mental images, with grounding, rather than the images controlling you. Elite athletes do it all the time, and it's a simple skill to learn.
- If a student is being deluged it can be useful to ask them who is in charge of their images and thoughts. Most students don't know, but given the opportunity to make up a solution I have heard "The MTV Controller", "The Conductor" and "The Features Editor" for example. Anything the students can relate to.
- There are useful tips in Chapter 7 to improve the organisation of mental images, so they don't become overwhelming.
- Relaxation is the key to reducing the chaos, which multiplies when EPIC students feel more stressed.
- We actually recommend tolerating students who fly off at a tangent – it enables them to make superfast connections, usually visual, gaining insights that others usually can't keep up with — a great skill for creativity.
-

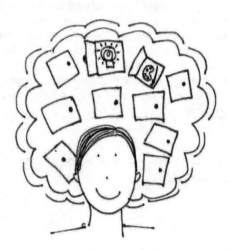

Sensory Overload

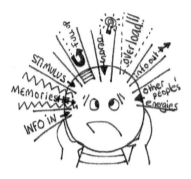

Symptoms:

- EPIC students will spend much of their time in sensory overload, using various strategies such as zoning out and stimming[37] to try to reduce the overload.
- EPIC students often live in their own world, do not pay attention in class and prefer to play alone
- They may exhibit an unusual attachment to toys. They may happily, obsess for hours, studying small objects like a row of toy cars, unconsciously switching off their peripheral vision.
- They can exhibit a similar obsession with patterns on cloth.
- Adults or children who are extremely ill can develop sensory overload symptoms, including withdrawal/closing-down when they are scared, as well as no speech, sleeping, eating, drinking, peripheral vision and hypersensitivity.
- Disrupted sleep pattern.
- Sensory issues (e.g. problems with an unexpected loud noise, certain materials, textures, wearing clothes, etc.).
- May become hyperactive/uncooperative/oppositional.
- Seem to hear sometimes but not others.

- May shun physical or eye contact.
- Hate being touched; sometimes a heavy grasp is better than a light tough, or visa versa.
- If you use a negative when you tell an EPIC student not to do something, they may do the opposite.
- Can develop normally and then start to disappear into themselves, before school age and be typically diagnosed as autistic.
- Being overwhelmed by thousands of pictures coming towards them and not being able to order or organise anything.
- Hate sitting still.
- The external world can cause sensory overload, but mental images can cause sensory overload even when the student is asleep.
- Disturbances in the gut.
- Massive invisible internal experiences.
- Students can cope at home but need medication to go to school. Some are the opposite coping better in school, which is very structured, than at home.

Topics to explore:

EPIC students live in continuous fear and anxiety that generates sensory overload, even when waking in a quiet environment. There are a host of reasons for their stress levels becoming too much. What may have started as stress is now a full-blown traumatic reaction, associated with significant fear and anxiety. You may only notice EPIC students in sensory overload, when they have external symptoms, like those itemised above. In addition, all the fear and safety issues may be generated internally and have few visible signs. In both cases, it is imperative that the students feel SAFE, in every aspect of life, from what they eat, where they live, their relationships, to going to school and releasing traumas.

Students can be born anxious and hyperactive or have developed this when they couldn't cope with a situation, such as neglect, adoption or simply going to school. When students feel unsafe, they have typically progressed past fight into flight – they want to run away from the situation or even run away from themselves. Of course, extreme frustration and anxiety, can quickly boil over into rage – "get me out of here!" as well as very challenging behaviour. Severe meltdowns as seen on the autistic spectrum will have a significant effect on memory and cause those all-important dendrites, used in memory, to wither.

Most people have no concept of how to control their mental images. These images are lovely when they are helpful but when unpleasant may create a state of recurrent trauma they would rather forget.

To escape this internal turmoil and fear, EPIC students will do any of the following to get out of sensory overload:

- Stimming - mostly repetitive movements the student can concentrate on while ignoring the rest of the world, such as rocking, lining up cars, tracing patterns, doodling or even fanatic drawing.
- Zone out the real world.
- Daydream or seem to be in a trance.
- "Be away with the fairies."
- Withdraw into themselves, to live in their own world.
- Not pay attention or concentrate.
- Runaway and jump about.
- Develop selective mutism.
- Even exhibit mental health problems (e.g. PTSD).

These can either be conscious or subconscious decisions. They are all responses for flight – get me out of here. I have known students to go blank when in sensory overload, and one said he just went down a black hole whenever it got too much, and after a break, a few minutes later, could come back.

Actions needed:

- Understand where the anxiety and fear come from by looking behind sensory overload to discover what is happening for that student, often visually.
- Practising grounding, mindfulness or meditation options.
- Don't stop stimming repetitive movements that calm the senses, until the students are relaxed enough to stop voluntarily.
- Start noticing when a student drifts off in class, and check what triggers this. They probably have their eyes raised, and they are simply watching a video, like Jimmy in Chapter 3.
- Don't touch someone in sensory overload until he has calmed down when you do touch, a firm grip is usually better than a stroke. The differences between your frequency and theirs can be very painful when stressed.

Ben's son was given up on by his school at the age of about 6, in the USA. Ben worked with his son for several years; his initial focus was to get him to come out of his own private world and join in with others. Ben did lots of very simple metaphors, stories, all encouraging Charlie to feel safe. Slowly Charlie decided to join in. Later, Charlie described perfectly the experience of leaving the world when in sensory overload and why "he had to act autistic then, to just reduce the overload." Having got him to come out, Olive coached Ben with all the visual literacy skills he needed. Ben now gets As and Bs and is preparing to go to college!

Jamie was in the hospital on ICU after a near-death traumatic experience, with sepsis. He seemed to be "going autistic." Although I know that current thinking makes this impossible, I witnessed him closing down, as he lost the ability to speak, eat, drink and sleep. I also knew that some parents had reported their child developing normally for a couple of years and then going backwards into themselves and being diagnosed as autistic. He could not be touched, without obvious chronic pain, and had lost his peripheral vision (he was fixated on the dots on his pyjamas) to reduce sensory overload. He had been running for two days in bed and then tried to make a run for it out of the hospital. I spent 14 hours helping him to feel safe again and again, and easing his delirium by releasing the trauma. After a good sleep (about 6 hours), he was back again, able to speak, eat, drink and communicate, and thankfully he recovered, knowing he was safe.

Literacy Affects so Many People

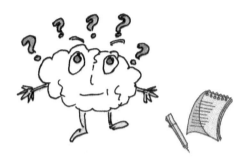

Symptoms:

In addition to what has been covered in Chapter 5:

- Reading levels are generally poor, and although phonics may have helped some, many EPIC students struggle with phonics, which individually don't have a visual meaning.
- Spelling is worse with many students because spelling phonetically just doesn't work in English.
- Students read slowly and don't remember what they read.
- Poor pronunciation.
- Speech and language problems. Some students need mental images of words in order to pronounce them.
- Likes listening to stories but has little interest in letters/words.
- Handwriting difficulties.
- Difficulty learning and using new words.
- Difficulties making up stories
- Gets words muddled up
- Much prefers reading from comics.
- Letters, p, q, b or d, move or rotate on the page, causing river effects and often jump off the page

- Students can read words they can't spell.

Topics to explore:

There is an old-fashioned term, "world blindness," which is used to mean that a person is unable to recognize and understand words that they see. This was the term used to describe dyslexia when it was first identified in the late 19th century. It means that the person does not seem to be able to remember the order and sequence of letters in a word from one time to the next. A student might be drilled for hours on an easy word, but the next time he saw the word, he would not recognise it. Such students are literally blind to the word; they are not picturing and storing words. Thanks to modern neuroscience, Empowering Learning™ can teach this skill quickly and easily, as an extension of the student's ability to create mental images. Applications for mental imagery such as literacy and numeracy are other **Elephants in the Classroom** – skills that experts take for granted but never teach children.

All good spellers will tell you they can see words in their mind's eye. It is quite odd when people say "I have to picture the word" as if it is some sort of deficiency.

Proof-readers spot typographical errors so easily because they can scan a page and mistakes just "jump out" at them because they are using the words in their Word Form Area for reference. Unfortunately, EPIC students who have no mental images of words can have all the words on a page jumping off the page and causing chaos.

Teaching mental imagery explicitly creates word recognition and accelerates any other reading programme.

Bright, exceptional, creative people are thinking differently, predominantly in terms of visualising pictures and have never thought of visualising words!

Many, who have letters flying around, use computer programmes/APPs to help with literacy. This is not a good strategy for those students who reverse letters and see them moving.

Using phonics programmes can accidentally, after many repetitions, cause students to develop mental images of words, so they become fluent readers.

If they are still using the frontal cortex for spelling, without accessing the Word Form Area, they won't spell accurately in English even if they can read the word. The reason for this is the orthographic depth of English. Mental images of homophones, words with silent letters and those that break the rules must be remembered visually.

"Insanity is doing the same thing over and over again and expecting different results." Misattributed to Albert Einstein, but nonetheless relevant.

No capital letter rotates and makes a different letter whereas p, q, b and d are all interchangeable in most fonts. That is also why most students prefer comics, as words are usually in capitals. Long words have more stability, although double vowels can switch.

We know that many EPIC students have developed excellent skills for pictures, but often have not developed the expertise to visualise words. In fact, 100% of people diagnosed with dyslexia whom other Empowering Learning™ Practitioners and I have met, have never developed these skills. But there is no reason why they shouldn't.

A mother of a child with Down syndrome once told me that Down syndrome students can't speak until they can visualise words. So, I checked with the Down Research Organisation, which confirmed this and I have also discovered that this can help with the speech of non-Downs students.

Annabel didn't have Down syndrome but mixed up some words, when speaking, and I guessed that the same technique might be worth a try. "Peace" and "place" were always a problem for her, so I got her to visualise them in different places, and she could immediately pronounce both of them - what a result!

Since then I have taught several speech therapists who have added picturing words to their toolbox of skills. There might be a much stronger relationship between mental images of words and pronunciation than we realise.

Odd things happen with words when you have not been taught how to visualise them:

Talking with Jim, a university lecturer, I asked him to picture a cat. Everything went well until he tried picturing the word cat. His image of the cat just "blew up" - paws, whiskers, tail, ears, and legs flying all over the place and a perfect example of how much stress words can generate. So we went back to pictures, re-assembled the cat and taught him grounding and relaxation, so he could then hold the word cat still.

Charlie, in a special needs school, said he could picture bits of words, but they were stuck to the inside of his forehead. I suggested he move them out 3-4 feet so he could get a better view. His face showed he saw something unpleasant so I enquired. He said he could see all the letters, but they were backwards. He then had to leave for his next class. When I saw him the following week, his words were all the right way around. The plasticity of the human brain is extraordinary.

Action needed:

- Offer the 7-point plan to any students who are struggling with literacy or numeracy.
- Increase safety, in all aspects of learning.
- Have students fix words on the page or in their mind's eye to stop them from moving, rotating, going fuzzy, running away or causing all sorts of distressing experiences.
- Make up stories that work with their strengths.
- Chapter 7 has a section on literacy and if you want to know more about improving literacy you can order a study guide from the resources section on www.empoweringlearning.co.uk.

Poor Numeracy

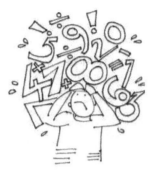

Symptoms:

- Topics like rotating images can be easy whilst algebra can be meaningless, e.g. 2x+3y.
- Teaching students to use number triangles without checking to see if they can visualise them.
- Difficulty remembering how numbers are written.
- Problems with estimating and counting.
- Poor memory for simple maths facts, like the area of a circle.
- Difficulties understanding mathematical symbols.
- Numbers reversed or rotated.
- Fast moving mental images can also encourage numbers and symbols to rotate, e.g. 6 turns into 9 and + into X.
- Problems counting backwards
- Problems remembering shapes.
- Confusion with similar looking numbers and directions, e.g. 92 or 29.
- Taking a long time to complete mathematical tables.
- There can be a lot of words in maths that will trouble poor readers.
- A hundred square and multiplication tables can put neurodivergent students into sensory overload.

Topics to explore:

There is an underlying problem with the way maths is taught in primary school; the curriculum assumes that you can picture numbers as mental images, under the age of 7. This is a presupposition of the whole system. For even the most basic mental arithmetic, mental images are essential; students need to be able to picture numbers, in any of their formats, as mental images. There is no alternative; this is after all what "mental arithmetic" means. People who are good at maths will tell you they can see numbers in their mind's eye. We should be checking every 4-5-year-old – it only takes seconds to check and minutes to teach the skill. Why don't we tell every parent and teach it as a simple "how to" skill that everyone can use? It can't do any harm.

EPIC students are thinking differently, predominantly in pictures and may never think of visualising numbers!

For those students who just know the answer without showing their workings out, grounding will help them slow down enough to articulate the calculation.

Actions needed:

Reduce anxiety about numbers, by teaching students how to visualise numbers in different forms, e.g. as dice, as counters, as numbers.

Teach algebra as a representation of an object, e.g. 6x + 4y can be thought of as 6 dogs + 4 cats. You can't make dogs into cats so x and y have to stay separate.

Times tables can be taught visually in any random order. Questions in maths are never in order.

For those who want to know "why," teach them the origin of numbers, in Chapter 7.

What Else Triggers Fear and Anxiety?

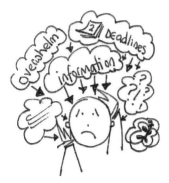

Fear and anxiety can be triggered by any of the previous stimuli and also all of the invisible sensory overloads. So, we have a loop here, a bit of stress magnifies into full-blown trauma that ungrounds the student, generating even more uncontrollable mental images that create more internal fear and anxiety. No wonder students withdraw into themselves looking for safety. Anxiety can come from many places. Many of which have nothing to do with the parents. For example:

- Pre-birth, including picking up on mother's anxiety and stress hormones through the umbilical cord.
- Post- birth, early adoption, Caesarean delivery, IVF, multiple pregnancy death, parental drug problems, not ready to be born (e.g. Induction, 2nd twin), energy separation.
- Trauma, fear, operations, identity trauma.
- Ungrounded family, not enough green space, vaccinations.
- Poor health, pain, operations, stomach upsets.
- Toxins, medication and environmental pollution.
- Busy environment.
- Going to school, being bullied.
- Being in frightening situations, feeling unsafe.

- Past life experiences.
- Over-reacting to situations – students may lash out and may feel no remorse.
- Not understanding a multitude of things in school, including why they are in trouble.
- When someone is incongruent.
- Poor sleep

With all of these your autonomic nervous system will be in sympathetic response, on high alert. This is the time when small things can magnify to trigger major explosions[38].

In addition to all these external triggers, there are also all the internal sensory overload factors which themselves generate even more fear and anxiety.

Incongruence is a big trigger for sensitive people, for example, telling the student he is good but they know you think the opposite. When students detect this, they will feel very unsafe and more anxious.

Your Gut

When you are anxious, this will be reflected in your gut. If your gut biome is not optimal, this will affect the function of your brain and your immune system and is often made worse by unhealthy eating, allergies, food intolerances, medication, toxins, etc.

The whole area of gut health is vitally important. There has been extensive research recently on the gut-brain connection. The gut plays a vital role in so many of the body's systems and transmits 400 times as much information to the brain than the brain transmits to the gut. This means when you have any disturbance in the gut microbiome, the brain is bound to be affected. It is not the remit here, but with some of the references attached, you will be able to investigate health improvements.

The movement into Functional Medicine and the mBraining initiative have amassed indisputable evidence about the effects on learning difficulties and many health issues.

Over-reaction to situations

EPIC students may over-react to situations, again causing sensory overload as they re-run previous bad experiences, which have the same emotional trigger and so they end up reliving the trauma visually.

In *Bridges to Success* see the story of Samual on page 27 about having no remorse.

Idioms and negatives

An idiom is a common word or phrase with a culturally understood meaning that differs from what its composite words' denotations would suggest. For example, an English speaker would understand the phrase "kick the bucket" to mean "to die" – and also to actually kick a bucket. Idioms present a significant challenge to many EPIC students. Reflecting on this through the lens of mental imagery, I realised what the problem is. Idioms are very visual, for example: Barking up the wrong tree.

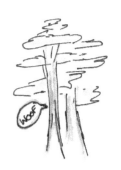

A hot potato	A penny for your thoughts
Actions speak louder than words	At the drop of a hat
Back to the drawing board	Ball is in your court
Cut corners	Be glad to see the back of
Beat around the bush.	Best of both worlds
Best thing since sliced bread	Bite off more than you can chew
Blessing in disguise	Burn the midnight oil
Can't judge a book by its cover	Caught between two stools
Costs an arm and a leg	Cross that bridge when you come to it
Cry over spilt milk	Curiosity killed the cat

Notice that none of these makes any sense to a highly visual EPIC student.

Jokes often have the same problem. There are also idioms in other languages.

Like idioms, EPIC students don't do negatives very well. For example, the command: "Don't stand up," focuses on a picture of standing up. "Sit down" would be a more successful instruction. Negatives are even more difficult to process when ungrounded and not accessing your internal dialogue.

A deluge of mental images

A deluge of mental images highlights some of the experiences of those on the autistic spectrum, where chaotic mental images are very common; even Temple Grandin talks about them.

For some EPIC students, their mental images lack clarity and any form of structure, and they are just deluged with all sorts of information. It is more comfortable to be in control of your images and not have them being in control of you. Some try to stop this chaos by stimming or having a manic desire to find patterns in everything. But this can become so 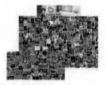 obsessive that they start looking for patterns even in the grass which would be overwhelming

When the student thinks of an essay to write, what happens? Instead of a few clear images, he may get hundreds of flashing images that eventually collect into a pile of junk. Alternatively, images may fly past so fast, they are good but don't stay long enough to allow him to write that essay. Or worse still, the pictures are so fast all you can see are black and white dots.

Picking up another person's energy

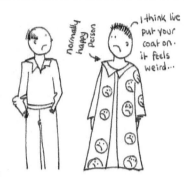

Do you have a friend who comes to see you when he is not in a good place? He may be fed up or tired and want a "shoulder to cry on," (notice the visual expressions here). When he has finished telling you how awful life is, how does he feel? How do you feel? He probably feels much better, which is why he came to see you. On the other hand, you probably feel a whole lot worse, having quite literally "picked up his stuff." Now that you are running his stuff, when you interact with someone else, are you responding as you or as your friend? EPIC students can pick up another person's energy and assume it is their own. For example, if a family member is sad, they may be sad too and they don't really know why. You will find more about this in *Bridges to Success* and Chapter 7 here. Running other people's energy can also exhaust you, and EPIC students, who are often ungrounded, will be very sensitive to this.

Empathy is the ability to experience the feelings of another person. It goes beyond sympathy, which is caring and understanding for the suffering of others. In my map of the world, empathy is unhealthy, as you are picking up another person's energy and unless you know how to let it go, running someone else's energy can make you sick. Doctors, dentists and counsellors often find themselves in this situation. For EPIC students who are having trouble keeping their own experiences under control the last thing they want is to be dealing with the emotions of others. It is said that many EPIC students can't feel empathy; it seems more likely that they are switching it off to avoid sensory overload.

Intuition

Intuition can be very upsetting for highly sensitive students. They may be confused as to whether they are seeing/hearing reality or hallucinating in some way. They may also mix up their thoughts and pictures with those of other people. Or they may not be listening to their intuition because their whole world is so noisy with overwhelming thoughts, they can't hear their own intuition, say about the right thing to do. You can imagine it like being at a noisy party and someone is trying to speak to you but you just can't hear them. You need space to calm down before having a chance to listen to your own wisdom. This is so vital when a meltdown grips you.

Human Eye Contact and Physical Eyesight

EPIC students will avoid human eye contact. One reason for this is that human faces change every second, causing instant overload. However, Thomas the Tank Engine[39], a popular toy with a face, has only one face which is much easier to comprehend and a dog has a few which is only a bit worse. When the EPIC student is less anxious and fearful, he will gradually be able to cope with more eye contact. However, notice how often EPIC students will look up when answering a question, this is their natural way of accessing visual information and shouldn't be discouraged.

It is worth mentioning some things about physical eyesight that may affect the student's mental images.

- If the student's physical eyesight is just restricted but clear, then don't assume that his mental imagery is poor. My experience is, in fact, the exact opposite. It seems that internal mental images get stronger to almost compensate for poor eyesight.
- Some students with extreme stress or sensory overload close down their peripheral vision to reduce their internal and external vision. Melvin Kaplan talks about specific evidence for the effects of stress on the development of central and peripheral vision and the connection with breathing patterns.
- Some students who typically use their peripheral vision regularly for, say, gaming and sport, may get a bit stuck in peripheral vision and not

understand how to close it down selectively, to reduce distractions when trying to concentrate. This does require a little practice.

Actions needed:

- The secret of controlling mental images is very simple: You just need to be calm and fully in your body, not anxious and ungrounded. The next chapter gives you simple tools to help others maximise the effectiveness of their mental images.
- Start chatting with students about the qualities of all these TV screens; for example, ask them whether they would like to turn some off.
- Try to create a sense of safety and comfort in their environment for students, so they:

  o Get out of flight, fight or freeze.
  o Are not frightened or overwhelmed by a whole host of things, including pre-birth/birth experiences, eating, going to school and even their own internal images.
  o Reduce the feeling of being overwhelmed caused by picking up other people's energies.

- Appreciate their high sensitivities:

  o To shunning physical and eye contact.
  o To different energies which can also scramble their energy and mental images

Understand that students may be frightened of new experiences. There are two time-orientated types of mental images: Those which are a memory of previous experiences and those which are formed through imagination. It seems that if you are flooded with the former, then the latter can be terrifying.

7.
Freeing Trapped Potential

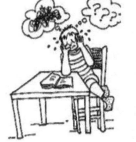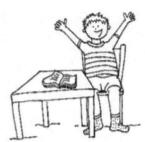

We have already examined the strengths of EPIC students in detail and discovered how mental images are enabling them to excel. In this chapter, we explore how to create the most effective mental images for the task.

No brain surgery is involved. All that is needed is a simple enquiry into the quality of someone's mental images and taking the time to coach him to find the easiest way to use them. As a source of on-going support, don't forget the Empowering Learning Facebook page.

As we saw in Chapter 5, there are just five simple topics that need to be addressed in more detail for those under 7: Creating Safety, Discovering Strengths, Getting Grounded, Controlling Mental Images, and Developing Visual Academic Skills.

Although these techniques are student-oriented, we recommend you try out as many as possible for yourself first. This will help you learn about your own experiences, and realise how we all learn differently. As a result, it may enhance your ability to teach others.

Safety First

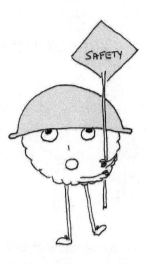

It is vital to create safety in everything students do – the last **Elephant in the Classroom** for this book. Some EPIC students can be so full of anxiety and fear that they would rather be alone in their own world and need coaxing to join our world. They also feel safer following the same (ritualistic) process, than doing anything that involves change.

Their fears can be very obvious; for example, being chastised for certain behaviours, being frightened of getting things wrong, tackling a new environment, being scared of certain foods and colours, or even just exhibiting continuous anxiety without any idea why they feel as they do. Everyone's anxiety will be different, from minor anxiety to full-blown trauma, so if you focus on praising what he is getting right, however small, as in Howard Glasser's Nurtured Heart Approach, he will start to work it out for himself.

It is important to look after your own state as well because if you are anxious students are likely to sense and feed off your anxiety too.

Growth Mindset and Validation

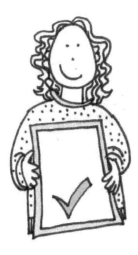

EPIC students who struggle with learning at school may begin to lose faith in themselves and their abilities. They may begin to link their learning differences with who they are: Their whole identity may become defined by perceived shortcomings. Some begin to see themselves as impaired rather than a wonderful, unique part of creation with many gifts and talents. Validation enables students to experience their intrinsic worth as human beings regardless of any challenges they are facing. For example, saying "You spent time checking your answers, well done! You got them all right," rather than the general "Oh, that's great," specifically points out the student's attitudes or actions and the positive impact they have had. We covered descriptive praise and growth mindsets in Chapter 4.

Differentiating between their self-concept and self-esteem can help students see possibilities. Self-concept is how you conceive of yourself in your essence, as a human being. Self-esteem is just a snapshot of your evaluation of how you are doing at a particular moment in time. So, if you are having a bad day, this may affect your self-esteem but not your overriding self-concept.

Validation is the next basic skill to learn. Have a go at the validation exercise for yourself.

- Ask your student to think about their positive qualities, what they have achieved to date and how they would have liked to have been congratulated.
- Ask them to imagine a symbol that represents all this and fill it up with all the unique ways they would like to be acknowledged and validated.
- When the symbol is full enough, top it off with glorious sunshine, so it gets even better.
- Be willing to open up to receiving all that is in the symbol and taking it with you.
- Notice how that feels.

These new perspectives are to help you let go of the stress that has been affecting you. They will also help you become even more successful with mental imagery and in many other aspects of your life. Hopefully, you will arrive at the point where you believe whatever you strive for is possible.

How to be Grounded

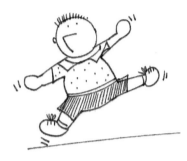 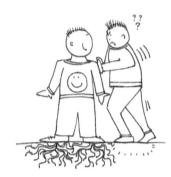

The object of getting grounded is to calm the nervous system, get it out of a sympathetic response and into a balanced or parasympathetic state.

One of the results of being anxious is to become ungrounded. In effect, a student "tries to run away" from the reality that is causing him so much distress. Grounding is all part of a young person's natural development and growth and you can see it in any group of children. Very young children run in a very bouncy, un-grounded way, with their legs flying all over the place. By the age of five to seven, most have learned to run more smoothly as they start to feel more grounded in themselves. As they grow up, they need to develop and experience their own sense of grounding. Sportsmen and women are often very grounded, although they may use different words to express this state. For example, grounding will help you to resist a rugby tackle, shoot penalties in football, convert tries in rugby, target shoot, and prepare to hit a golf ball.

Being born to grounded parents gives students an experience of grounding at a very young age. When we are born, we can ground through our parents who carry us about, and we can continue to ground like this for some time. If parents are very un-grounded, however, students may struggle to get that experience for themselves and hence will have much more difficulty in developing it naturally. A child who comes into the world in a very traumatic pregnancy or birth may never feel comfortable on the planet, from their earliest days and have extreme difficulty settling to being grounded. Fortunately, grounding is a skill you can easily learn.

Grounding is a very basic feeling that enables you to feel comfortable in your own body, more relaxed, centred and balanced. There are thousands of ways that grounding will improve your health and wellness. A typical symptom of being ungrounded is to feel a bit wobbly or unbalanced in certain circumstances. For instance, to stand on one leg, we have to ground through the other, or we fall over.

A simple way for students to achieve grounding in seconds, without others noticing, is:

- Stand up, think of all the things you have to do in the next few hours and notice how distracted or stressed you feel. Are you wobbly?
- Now bring your attention to the soles of your feet. Think of a tree, imagine you too have tree roots growing out of your feet, right down into the centre of the earth and spreading right out so however hard you are pushed you won't fall over. (This is also a useful skill for the playground.)
- This is known as your grounding chord, make it big enough for a football say. You can connect one or more to your feet, the base of your spine, your heart, the centre of your head; anywhere you feel needs grounding.
- If you are feeling stressed, breathe in for two and out for six a few times. You can imagine blowing out a candle or blowing a few bubbles from one of those bubble tubes; both can help to achieve this 2-6 breathing. Now that you are balanced you can return to breathing in for a count of four and out for the same, to maintain balance. Walking or tracing a labyrinth can also help your left-right brain balance.

- Relax into your feet and imagine releasing any stress into the ground through your roots on the out-breath. Then imagine bringing all the earth's nutrients and strength up into your body on the in-breath. (You might like to think of the metaphor of seed germinating and growing into a plant; gaining energy from the ground and releasing waste products.)
- Notice how many thoughts are running around in your head, all competing for attention. Take your consciousness down into your belly and after about 30 seconds, notice how the number has reduced.
- Keep releasing until you feel totally stable, "present in your body" and "solid," with little or no thought traffic.
- With a little practice, you can do this equally well sitting down, with your arms and legs uncrossed and your feet flat on the floor.

I find an old-fashioned egg-timer invaluable. As you watch the sand pass through, you can gradually become more and more grounded. If you have a child in sensory overload, give him an egg-timer and if he turns it over it is your cue to stop talking and leave him a minute or two to re-ground.

Another tip for grounding is to run the palm of your hands together and then rub your face. You will see people doing this subconsciously when they are stressed. I even have a pack of 52 cards that each have a different way to get grounded[40], complete with ideas for children. I often let students choose a card and see how that resonates for them.

Grounding may trigger emotions the student is trying to get away from, out of conscious awareness. So, you and the student need to learn how to get grounded and release blocks until an optimum learning state is achieved.

There are many metaphors or techniques you can use to achieve this state; I have included others in *Bridges to Success*. You can also ground a room, because being ungrounded is very catching between students. See what works best for you!

Here is a picture of some of the more unusual ways people try to get grounded – disconnecting their body from their head, grounding outside your body (disassociated), grounding through a channel that is too thin (unbalanced), pushing all their emotions down into their legs (blocked) and jumping/climbing around to avoid the ground (flying high). It can be very interesting to ask students how they are trying to ground today.

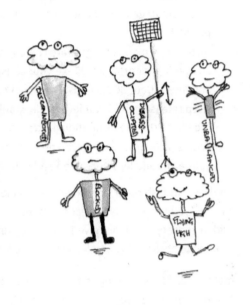

A child who wants to be grounded unconsciously you may see disappear under a pile of blankets, cushions or even be addicted to a trampoline.

There are many physical exercises to help with grounding, originating from body work, chiropractic practice, yoga, craniosacral massage and primary reflexes. Physical products such as weighted (or even a pile of heavy) blankets, using a wobble cushion or a squeeze machine can all assist. The movement of a safe swing can often also calm the nervous system. Even following the lines in a labyrinth can assist right/left brain integration.

This section has given you several options as different students will find particular ideas better than others.

Releasing Blocks and Scary Pictures

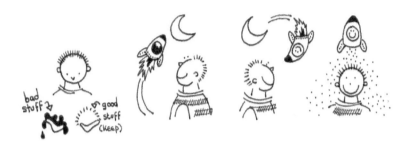

Some EPIC students have real problems getting grounded, running into blocks of some sort. Some students have been ungrounded from birth and are most likely to run into blocks which is the reason they may spend so much time getting away from being grounded. Here is a metaphor we use for releasing blocks or scary pictures and again you can make up your own.

Invite the student to consider the fastest thing he can think of; choosing a rocket ship for example. Ask him to put the stuff he doesn't want in the rocket ship and send it off to the other side of the moon. Then invite the student to picture another rocket ship coming back from the moon, full of confidence and all the things he wants to achieve. Have him shower this on his head. How does he feel now? You will often see a beaming smile. Remember you can change the contrst, clarity, colour, encase them in a wall of glass, ground out any energy; anything that helps the student. You are the sovereign of your own energy field.

There are many other metaphors you can use. There are a number in *Bridges to Success* or you can make up your own. Emotional Freedom Technique (EFT) is also a well-known technique for releasing emotions. I especially like the positive statements.

The Basic Qualities of Mental Images

Once the student is grounded, you can investigate the qualities of his mental imagery. By focusing on entering the student's map of the world, you can help him to explain his experience of images and guide him to make it as comfortable as possible. Discussing students' strengths is a great way to talk about their images. Later in this chapter, I will discuss slowing the deluge of too much information, but for now, let's cover the basics.

Mental images may simply be in the wrong place, causing the student a great deal of confusion. As mentioned, they can be too close, too far away, stuck in movies, fractured, flipped by 90, 180 or 270 degrees, too bright, too dark, transparent, solid, too many objects on one screen, too many screens. You can discuss with a student these simple qualities and help them move them around until they are in the most comfortable position for him, which is likely to be just above head level with eyes slightly raised to the left or the right. When grounded he should be able to choose how many screens and whether they are still or movies. Many EPIC students are often in very fast-moving videos, reflecting their very fast brains. Help them to play with the images they get and use grounding to help them obtain conscious control.

Some people can create glorious multi-colour pictures like a high definition TV; others get black and white pictures, others get cartoons, and some may just know what something looks like but can't really "see" it. All of these are fine, and like so many things, if you start to pay more attention to them, they get clearer.

Students can and do have very different experiences. They need to capture a good image so that they can retain it. If the student is certain he doesn't have pictures, it is probably his expectations that are letting him down. Try the following and don't be too serious. Request the student:

- To look at something simple like an apple, pet, house, front door for instance and really study it. Then see if he can recall it, with his eyes open or closed.
- Next, you could have him try a favourite TV programme or a film scene.
- Tell him to look into something really lovely like a perfect flower or the picture of a lovely scene (use the picture that pops up on your computer when you start it up). Study it in detail for several minutes and then see if he can recall any of it.
- If he is really stuck, recall a minor disaster, like the dog or the cat being sick on the carpet, or the car getting damaged. This often jolts the memory into realising that it does have pictures, and you can work with him from there.

Help him to develop pictures from there. Alternatively, he may have such fast pictures that he can't keep them still to look at, e.g. he just "knows" what colour his car is, but doesn't see a still image. Of course, some people have nasty images and should use the simple "releasing blocks" exercises to get rid of those.

Working with one 8-year-old EPIC student, I asked him if he could picture a cat. He said yes, and whilst looking forward towards me he pointed behind him and said, "It's over there in the cupboard behind the blue curtain." I enquired whether that was a convenient place and he said, "No, I can't see it very well." I then asked whether I could move it and brought it round in front of him. He was very happy with the new position and could then describe the cat in detail, saying, "That's a lot better. I can see it now."

Practice to get Better Pictures

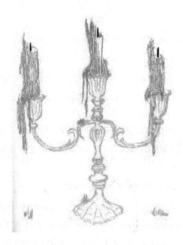

Mental imagery is normal, just like breathing. How do you find your way home or recognise your family members? Part of the successful recall of images is to be able to take a good "picture" of something you want to recall, noticing any details. For instance, if you lose a bunch of keys, you may not have an image. Next time you put your keys down, take a picture in your mind of where you left them, complete with the background. When next you are on the hunt, recall that picture in your mind, and you will find your search easier. Whenever you are looking for something, just picturing it will assist you. In addition, taking a picture of, for example, locking the front door before you leave and where you parked the car will help your memory.

There was a recent TV programme on Channel 4, in the UK, called How to Improve Your Memory. Three celebrities were taken through two visual memory techniques. Gok Wan said that his memory was only full of fashion and he had not done well in school. He learnt how to remember the whole periodic table plus various related facts and finished with the best score of all. There are lots of visual memory skills, you can try out that have been developed by those with astounding memories.

Creating Imaginary Pictures

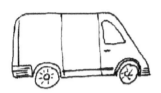 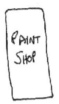 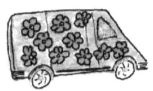

Some EPIC people have exceptional skills for recalling information they have seen before, going back years in minute detail, but they have difficulty imagining new information or picturing the future. We postulate that this is because they are so used to being able to picture places and things they have seen before. By contrast, new places can be terrifying and creating goals for the future can be difficult.

Working from the student's strengths, you can guide a student to create new imaginary pictures, known as visual constructs, from an amalgam of recalled pictures. Try this way of transforming from the familiar to the unfamiliar. Picture a van driving into a paint shop or a car wash if you prefer. It goes in yellow and accidentally gets painted bright blue, and it is covered with flowers. Notice how the van looks. Now you have created a new unique van in your imagination. Notice the use of the language, "picture" works well for recall and "imagine," once he is confident, is better for creating visual constructs.[41]

Intuition

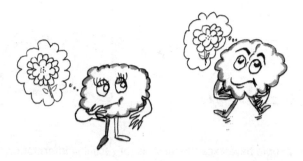

If students are very sensitive, they can certainly pick up on other people's emotions, especially close family members. In addition, they may pick up on someone else's emotions and start to get swamped by them. The recipient may even start to behave like the other person, spreading emotions like sadness and misery to those they meet.

Clairvoyance enables students to "pick up" on your pictures, so if you want to introduce someone to a new concept, it can be useful if you imagine it and see if that helps them to reduce any anxiety. Clairsentience is the expression used for people who seem very insightful, just know something without knowing how they know – parents will realise when this happens. Many EPIC students are clairvoyant and/or clairsentient.

The simple techniques above, for energy clearing (including all the pictures students are holding), grounding and releasing blocks, enables students to enjoy their intuition without being overwhelmed by it.

Controlling Mental Images

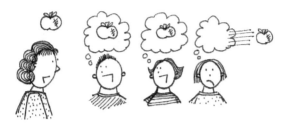

Controlling mental images is as simple as controlling your breath and, with a little practice, it can be perfected. EPIC students need to be in control of their images, not the other way around. For example, if they want fast-moving images for creative work, that is their choice, but when they get distressed in sensory overload, they want to be able to slow things down.

The first thing a student needs is to learn is how to control images through calmness, relaxation, becoming grounded and being entirely in his body. Fortunately, this can be achieved in seconds, as even small things may stress him out, and he may not have time for meditation. The student needs to be calm and alert. This is an optimal or effective learning state and can be achieved quickly and easily through grounding. Although mindfulness and meditation techniques are great, speed is essential when a student becomes stressed. Once the student has learned to become grounded, mental images are much easier to control and develop.

A state is only a definition of how you are at any particular time; so being on your mark for a big race you may be grounded. By contrast, when you are struggling in the last stages you may be ungrounded, and when trying to read you may be in a completely different state. Developing metaphors or stories is the best way to help students. The next few pages give you examples of stories; you are welcome to personalise them for the student.

Slowing Down the Student's Brain

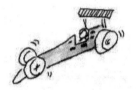

Ask the student to imagine his brain is a car and what sort of a car would it be? Would it be a Formula 1 racing car or something much slower like Trotter's 3-wheel van from *Only Fools and Horses*[42]?

In our experience, all EPIC students have something like a Formula 1 racing car, and occasionally they also add, "… but it is stuffed with cotton wool!" To have a fast-moving brain is a great skill, but you need to be able to take control like any driver, and apply the brakes when necessary? You need wheels to connect to the ground, brakes to drive at the appropriate speed, driving lessons to be effective in all circumstances. Again, students need skills to get grounded and they must learn skills to control their own brain and imagery.

John loved watching motor racing and unsurprisingly had difficulty keeping up with his very fast brain and getting grounded. I suggested he imagine going around a track and stopping in the pit lane. You could see him desperately trying to stop his imagination in the pits, but every time he couldn't hold the image still. It took him 4 laps, knocking over lots of imaginary people before he finally came to rest at the red light. He looked relieved that he had managed to stop his very fast brain, because he now had a choice.

There are lots of meditation techniques to help you slow-down a very busy brain. Lorraine E Murray's Calm Kids has this focus.

Reducing the Deluge

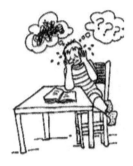 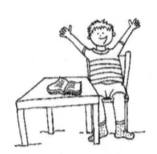

Again, grounding is the first step to reducing the deluge, and then organisation is the second. But more importantly, exploring who is in charge of this deluge of mental images, may enable the student to converse with that part. Grounding or mindfulness will allow the student to slow down the deluge of information his brain is providing, and he may need to release more blocks as he makes progress. Take it gently as this habit may have been built up over months and years, and it may be a shock to release it.

> Jimmy was 12 years old and had masses of mental images, 24-7. I asked him who was in charge of them and he looked dumbfounded, "I have no idea," was his instant reply. So I asked him whom he would like to put in control and he said, "Well there is the MTV controller." So I asked him whether he thought that would work well. He nodded and looked deep in thought for a few minutes. Then a big smile broke out as he said: "That's better, we now have a programme schedule for the whole day."

We have met cases where all this barrage of information is below eyeline. All this mass of pictures appears on any topic, when they look down, and the images are out of control. At the same time, they are not very clear, the student just knows the pictures are there, and if only he had some structure, he could use them. Again, too many fast pictures will increase sensory overload.

Although for some this may be an autistic-like symptom, you don't need to be on the autistic spectrum (ASD) for this to occur[43]. Ask the student to notice where the torrent is starting and going to. Perhaps it is coming straight for them from the front or just skirting around them. If it is triggering negative reactions, it is likely to be very close. Well, they can move it. Try sending the torrent back against the wall opposite and raising it up to just above eye level. See it coming from one side and disappearing to the other. Hopefully, all this activity is now out of their space. How do they feel now?

A lady came to see me once with a challenge of not being able to make decisions for anything in life from what to cook for dinner to what clothes to wear. She had no diagnosed learning difficulty. Not knowing why she couldn't do this, I asked her if she could give me an example. She said she could never make her mind up about what to cook for dinner; she got completely overloaded and gave up - this irritated her husband until he took charge. I asked her what mental images she had. Clearly, no one had ever asked her this before and after a few seconds, she said, she had hundreds of pictures flying towards her from the bottom right in her visual field with loads of things to eat. I got her to get grounded and then asked her to organise them on a sort of imaginary wall planner, blue-tacking all the images she wanted onto the planner and then making the best selection. She was looking up and going from left to right, so they didn't come straight towards her. She quickly started reorganising, and when she came back the next week, she said she now had spaces for recipes and ingredients for any meal she wanted to make. What a result in just 15 minutes of exploration. With the help of a virtual wall planner, she could stand back and see the options, she could generalise from this to other decisions in her life.

As a learning coach or parent, this will sharpen up the student's sensory acuity – his ability to notice what someone else is experiencing. Notice the student's eyes when he is telling you a story or recounting an event. A student with a good recall will invariably be looking up seeing mental images and just speaking about what he sees. If you want to ask a question, make it a visual one, not an auditory one, as this is likely to knock him off track, and he may even have to start the explanation again. If he has multiple screens, his eyes are likely to be darting about. You can ask his brain to change any of the qualities of the images and see what happens. Give his brain a simple metaphor to help:

- When you want to concentrate on one particular task you may want to turn off all but one screen; try imagining a remote control that enables you to select which channel to focus on.
- When you are trying to get to sleep, you may want to dim the brightness, for example.

It may be beneficial for most students also to learn to type without looking down, to keep them in their visual field.

Phil was a bright teenager but couldn't get focused on writing essays. I decided to check out what happened to his mental images when trying to write about World War II, for example, He just saw a pile of rubbish in front of him on the floor – no structure, no organisation. We worked on increasing focus on just one part of the essay: "asking" all the other topics that were not World War II to leave his space. A useful metaphor was when he is in a history lesson, and the teacher has booked the room, all the French and German classes need to keep out, it is not their space. Then I suggested he break the task down into sections, so he decided on military planes first. With a touch of grounding, he generated a single screen in his visual field and started loading up pictures of planes. Having organised his thoughts like this, he could identify what he wanted to say. When he went into the next topic I asked him what he wanted to do with the planes, and he looked at me, in disbelief and said, "Just wipe them away with a windscreen wiper," and they were all gone. He was pleased to have gained control of all these pesky little pictures.

This may have been the first time he had space in his head for 13 years! We then brought in the tanks and managed to drill down into some of the tank details. He kept looking down. I asked him to look up and see just one tank. There was nothing there. He had created space again. Slowly we tried to move one tank up into his visual field. He didn't think he could see it, but he could describe it.

Conclusion: All his V has been in K, maybe from birth, causing major sensory overload. His head-banging, at a younger age, was his only way of trying to get this stuff that he wasn't really conscious of under control. I am hopeful he can get the big picture (maybe by looking down) and then develop the details by looking up.

Organising Chaotic Mental Images

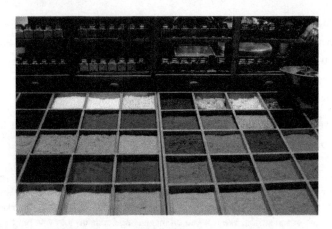

Now that our EPIC students have gained a bit of control over their mental images, let's add a bit of structure that works for them.

Many people experience overwhelming mental images; for example, they will describe "the very mention of a word like shoes, and I am overwhelmed with hundreds of pictures of shoes. It is like a snowstorm, and they are all coming straight for me, all different shapes, sizes, designs and colours." Autistic students are not meant to be able to generalise, but as their subconscious can shower them with loads of different shoes, it seems more likely that they can generalise but prefer to avoid generic words to reduce the overload. A tip for parents would be to say, "Can you find your blue shoes?" Try to be as specific as possible.

The coach needs to be careful not to be judgmental about images that seem a bit "crazy." Offer the student a choice and work with him until he is more comfortable. See if he can create structure.

What Organisation Works Best for You?

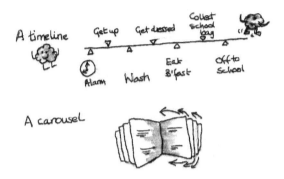

Now, ask the student: How would you like to organise your mental images? When he is calm, relaxed and grounded, have him play with different organisations and just come up with something that works for him. There are a number of possibilities:

A timeline of facts, to organise past, present and future events, from left to right, could be great for say, history revision.

> I met Jim, an estate agent at a local networking event. He told me how he organised details of every house he had for sale. All the details were in his mental imagery and organised in a sort of vertical carousel. When looking for properties with specific characteristics or locations, he could just flick through each one in his mind's eye.

Students can have personal time lines for organising themselves. He can imagine a day or a week like using a wall planner for critical events, so he can step back and see the bigger picture, disassociated from it. This is good when dealing with a hectic schedule or something unpleasant. Alternatively, the student can have a timeline that goes through him; future in front of him, present in him and past behind him. The disadvantage of this arrangement is that you can get clogged up behind you whilst it is difficult to see past the next event into the future. The advantage is that you are really associated into it, and thus fully able to feel emotions.

Learning Applications for Mental Images

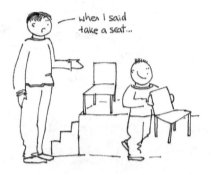

At Empowering Learning™, we have pieced together a great deal of information from research and neuroscience, to enable students to quickly and easily learn how to use their strengths in mental imagery for all sorts of applications, including spelling, reading, maths, comprehension and memory.

This is the area in which Empowering Learning's™ Jumpstarting Literacy and Numeracy programme has been a world leader for many years. For details go to www.empoweringlearning.co.uk and read *Bridges to Success*. It is a simple skill that practitioners with this expertise, teach in minutes.

"This is so easy, isn't it cheating" A 9-year-old boy in Holland

If a student has obsessions, you need to enter his obsession with him. If you don't, he will not be interested. So, if you are teaching a child to spell, who is obsessed with Thomas the Tank Engine, for example, get him imagining all the words on the sides of the trucks.

Be careful with the English language as it has so many idioms, EPIC students will take them very literally.

Mental Images of Words

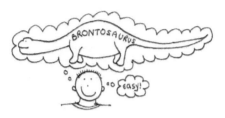

Students who think in the big picture (i.e. the whole word for literacy) can then fit in the phonemes, whereas they find it difficult to rely on a purely auditory strategy to build up from phonemes to whole words, along with all the quirks of the English language. Although phonics is the accepted norm for teaching literacy, the last phase of phonics should be to move to word recognition for fluent reading. So teaching mental imagery in parallel can speed up this process and at the same time, be a vital tool for spelling, comprehension, handwriting, maths and concentration. It isn't phonics or mental imagery; it is both for fluency and depends on the language.

Occasionally, I meet a student who has bits of words missing. These can be, for example, pieces missing out of the middle or from either end. Bits missing out the middle are quite common and are best explained by someone reading with left eye dominance and then changing to right eye dominance around the middle of the word. Most people cope with this well, but some just lose letters.

Reading aloud can be a dauting task as you feel you are going to be judged for any mistakes. Try reading to a young child or a dog - they won't worry about any mistakes and dogs create a feeling of calmness and grounding.

Just for fun you can try some Chinese and Japanese characters. It is really essential that you visualise these.

Paul came to see me with his younger brother, and Paul explained how his spelling had dramatically improved when he was younger. He was now an estate agent presenting lots of information about people's properties without any sign of dyslexia. I chatted to him about people's different experiences of mental images, recalling one teenage boy I had met at a bookshop signing who came up on his own to ask me why he couldn't picture words correctly, saying he only got the middles. I asked him where his mental images were. They were on the end of his nose. I put my hand up where they were and gently walked backwards to about 6 feet, raising my hand up a little. He was so excited, exclaiming, "I can see the whole word now, Thank you. I have got to go and tell my friend." Suddenly Paul said, "I know what happened. It was like words were stuck on the inside of my crash helmet. I could only see the middles; all the other letters were wrapped around the side of my head."

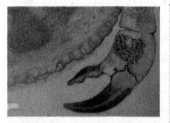

Willow is one of the very few clients to have completed her intake form saying that she could visualise words but couldn't spell, so I asked her what her images looked like. She explained that the middle of the word was often missing. She was visualising straight ahead, so I explained the problem with this and suggested she try to the left or the right and count how many letters she had in each position. She decided that up to the left was the clearest and she could immediately spell all the words. She was 16, an exceptional artist, and only a few months away from taking her GCSEs.

"My sons have both been diagnosed with Asperger's and ADHD. Since learning the Empowering Learning™ visualisation techniques, the changes in the boys have been remarkable. After six years of constant battles and resistance to the concept of having to have to sit down to learn words, there is now no reluctance to participate in the learning. This in itself is a great relief and very welcome.
Words are being learnt, remembered and recalled in a relaxed and easy manner, gone are so many of the frustrations. Both boys have progressed from being willing only to learn an agreed six words from the school spellings list to the full list of twenty and as such now participate fully with the rest of their class. I am so pleased and amazed at the progress that they have made, These simple but powerful techniques have certainly been keys to unlocking this area of learning for them and help me keep calmer too." Emma

Mental Images of Numbers

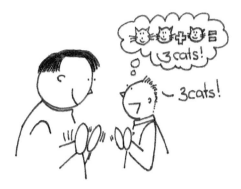

The way numeracy is taught, it presupposes that students can visualise numbers in all their formats, for example as counters, on dice, as numbers.

It is really useful to understand why the numbers are the shapes they are. Mathematicians in the ancient world created the original set of algorithms to represent the number of angles each shape had. The stars indicate the angles in each number. The original number set didn't have a zero; this was added later with no angles. So 4 has 4 angles, 8 has 8 angles and so on. Students with good visual recall may find this assists students to add up.

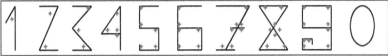

Visualising numbers is the same as visualising letters and words. Once visualising words has been mastered, try adding numbers to help the student master this skill too. Copy '2cats' and '6eggs' onto Post-its and ask the student to try visualising these, in the same way as they do words. You might also like to try the two "text speak" words "nice2cu" and "gr82cu". There is more information on mathematics in our study guides, such as how to visually learn times tables.

Memory and Comprehension

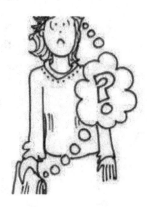

Mental images are, of course, vital to memory.

Some people know they have a photographic memory, but don't let your expectations of perfect pictures hold you back.

Sometimes students say they don't seem to have a good memory. This is more often about whether they are interested in the topic. For visual people to remember the information, they can learn how to make it into a single picture or a story, with a series of pictures, even for a simple shopping list.

Comprehension is another visual skill. The easiest way to remember what you read is to create a mental image at the end of every sentence or paragraph. You can also string together these images into a video and then just run the video to recall the events.

To improve comprehension, start with finding an audio recording of a very graphic story, like *Alice in Wonderland*. Listen to the story and make up pictures to remember what you have heard. If you are reading to a young child, you can take any story and add a few prompts to help trigger his memory – this is like stage management for the brain. In this example, the brackets [ ] indicate the stage management instructions: There were lots of tin soldiers marching along the road [suggest that the child should attempt to notice how many, how many per row, how many rows]. They were wearing blue and silver uniforms, with a black stripe up the trousers, [tell him to put that in his picture]. As they came past, a teddy bear was marching with them. He was wearing a blue uniform and a silver cap [add the bear to the picture].

Now that the student has a picture of everything, he has heard he will be able to answer questions about the pictures he has created in his mind's eye.

As the student's reading improves, he will be able to read and create pictures at the same time, without any prompts. Comprehension will automatically become easier.

I met Brian in a café. He was a dyslexic racing driver, who didn't understand how he had become so successful, so quickly. He had brilliant mental images of the track, and I asked if he could practice going slow to take better pictures. His face said it all, "I'm a racing driver I don't do slow," but he did agree it might be good to run around the track before a race to get better pictures. After he got grounded, he could read the menu and order his dinner – a completely new experience for this dyslexic.

Conclusion: Creating your own Map

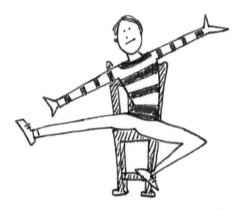

I should like to tell you a storey about Freddy:

> Freddy, a bright child goes to school – how do the parents know he is bright? Because he is creative, charming, and a bit of a character.
>
> Freddy's parents never did well at school; mum has become an artist, and dad somehow got into IT and became a successful engineer. They notice that Freddy doesn't seem to be enjoying school, and by the time he is 6 years old, he is miserable about school. He is complaining every morning about a stomach ache and pleads with his mother to keep him at home. When he does go, he will often be in tears and, by the end of the day, is exhausted when he comes out of school.
>
> Freddy has also had more than his fair share of discussions with the headteacher and the special needs advisor, for behavioural issues – frustration boiling over, inattention and conflict with other children.
>
> The school is very supportive, but the teachers don't understand why he is struggling. Although he has friends at school, he can't seem to make any progress with reading and spelling.
>
> His mother is getting more anxious, as he never sits still, and his letters and numbers are the wrong way around. However, the school said that lots of children do this and they grow out of it.

His father keeps saying, "Don't worry I found reading difficult until I was about 30 and then it suddenly seemed to make more sense. I battled through and got a good job; you will be fine. It was like a switch had gone on in my brain; I am sure you will get it too."

As Katy, his younger sister grows up, she is reading very well before the age of 4. Freddy is still struggling and by this time, his friends are racing ahead. By now Freddy is feeling extremely bad about himself and losing hope. He says "I am stupid," and, "I don't want to live like this." As you might expect, those words upset and frighten everyone.

Mum and Dad start to believe that Freddy has inherited this and their guilt grows too; he is pressing their buttons every day as they see him struggle as they did. They even feel guilty praising Katy.

How many students like Freddy do you know?

Freddy has now been assessed by the school as dyslexic, which in part is a relief. On the other hand, his parents hate the label, but they hope he will get more help. However, not much seems to change, and over the years they are told that school budget cuts make it very difficult to help further. Mum and Dad realise that he is excellent at some things, especially music and sport (**misunderstood greatness**), but they are so busy and upset dealing with the hell of daily homework for them to really notice. Freddy has developed a twitch, often zones out and suffers frequent meltdowns over relatively trivial things that he doesn't seem to be able to understand. Even the simplest written work is a no-go area. His behaviour is getting worse. He is permanently distracted in school and his "friends" are starting to tease him.

He is very good at his PlayStation, and seems quite addicted. He has an excellent imagination for making up stories but can't write them down. By contrast when it comes to construction toys like Lego, he can do them even without the directions.

The school is very accommodating and the latest Ed. Psych report identifies dyslexia, ADHD and maybe slight Asperger's and dyspraxia. He has had various tests for hearing, sight (letters on the page were moving) and behaviour and now wears those pink tinted glasses – which he hates. They seem to help, but you can imagine what the other kids say. He is dropping further and further behind, and his behaviour is deteriorating.

When he enters secondary school at the age of 11, he is very articulate and has become the "class clown." Despite his appalling literacy, he has excellent math skills, but his writing is illegible. He is very thin (his diet is not good) and wobbly and he also has a wheat intolerance. Moreover, he has regular meltdowns and has earned quite a reputation, having spent much time in the headteacher's office over the last year.

How many Freddy's do you know?

At the age of 16 he was permanently excluded for the latest classroom prank in a long series of disruptive behaviours. This one went wrong, and a child was hurt badly. Even Freddy was very upset about what had happened to his friend, so he ran out of school and jumped the perimeter fence into the street. So now the school has a safeguarding issue too.

This is where I came in.

At 16 years old: **Misunderstood greatness**, unrecognised talents, low self-esteem, almost no literacy, inability to concentrate, terrible handwriting, ongoing depression, and a realisation "this was the end of the road." Out of school with no qualifications. His next stop was probably as a young offender. What had gone so very wrong?

Enter the whole family plus the special needs co-ordinator, all very stressed with his mother close to tears. She was at the end of her tether.

I taught them to start relaxing, to release the stress and to get themselves grounded, fully in their bodies.

I checked to see who could see words in their mind's eye. Dad said yes but gave up when the words were longer than 5 letters. Katy saw perfect words; mum had no concept, and Freddy's mouth dropped open as if he had been shot. He exclaimed "**This is Instagram for the brain.**" He clearly had no idea that this was possible and was just a little angry that no one had told him before that this was what he should be doing.

After teaching them all to get grounded, paying particular attention to their sensory systems. I taught them how to get their visual images under control and how to visualise words accurately. This all took about 60 minutes and Freddy was engaged in the first non-maths lesson for the first time in years. Mum and Dad agreed, "**This makes so much sense**, I now understand."

Talking with Freddy about how he did maths, we had great visual images of numbers but he had never thought of using the same skill for words.

I then taught him to let go of all that negativity he had picked up over the years plus the energy that accompanies it, because now he had a new skill. He was going to be able to learn much more easily, and he might even understand some of the lessons he had zoned out in over the years. I also taught him to catch the awful feeling when he was en route to a meltdown and let that go before it overwhelmed him and how to deal with busy environments.

He looked as if he would have been happy to stay there practising all afternoon, but it was time for swimming so off he went with the broadest grin you have ever seen on a 16-year-old.

How many students like Freddy do you know who might achieve this with just 60 minutes of tutoring?

Two weeks later a different family walked in. They were all much more relaxed, Freddy had been given individual lessons outside school hours by his favourite teacher, the Rugby coach, who had always known Freddy had great potential if he could only tap into it. He had now discovered the **elephant in the room**, which was well known in sports – mental imagery. Freddy had achieved astonishing results. He now:

- spent time every day practising
- read quite fluently even with expression
- spelled 7 letter words
- improved his handwriting
- decreased his exhaustion
- suffered no meltdowns
- started eating better and even a little bread
- had cut out all the junk food.

Having a special needs co-ordinator, there had been a real boost:

- she had organised the extra lessons to help him catch up
- the school had promised he could take the exams.

She was now getting fired up and confident enough to launch a **mental imagery revolution in her school** for all the 11 year olds entering.

Freddy, being **neurodivergent** started to see the situation differently. He was good at maths, so decided to add up the cost of all the special attention he had commanded over the years. There were 10 years of support from learning assistants, special needs time, head teachers' time, at least 10 assessments he could remember and special glasses, amounting to £56,000. If he had gone on to college, he could have received a disability student allowance a further £65,000 over 3 years to support him in class. His calculations didn't take into account the stress on the whole family, the time his parents needed to take off from work and any support he would need when he left education. Now he was **freeing his trapped potential** and excited about his future.

He then calculated that for those who went to college, it was more than £100,000 each. He saw a report recently that there are 600,000 students currently in education with SpLD, let alone those without labels who are underachieving. This is an enormous strain on the country when such simple skills can easily be taught in primary school. In both the UK and the USA it is estimated to be more than 10% of all children

Freddy's story has many similarities to my own. However, I grew up in a different age where you just kept plodding along, hoping things would get better and being controlled to be "good," even if school and homework were exhausting and time-consuming. The word "dyslexia" wasn't known in my school, and I don't think it had even been invented then. My saving grace was being really good at sports, something my school offered me every day and on weekends. I left school without all the A levels I needed to get into university, but I was miraculously given a place to study maths by my delightful professor. I will always be indebted to him.

A Collaborative Initiative

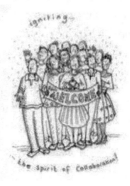

So now that you are becoming experts in mental imagery, we all need to work to empower parents and teachers with skills they didn't know they needed. Imagine for a moment if we could integrate these simple skills into the educational curriculum for our students in their first years at school. Imagine what it would be like for all students to have the skills to learn more easily and avoid their deepening confusion. Imagine happier, more confident students, reduced financial costs and less emotional stress on parents and schools, not to mention improved results, less frustration and conflict, fewer offenders, the list goes on. Imagine how much that would change our classrooms, homes and communities. Isn't this a challenge worth taking, a prize worth fighting for? Imagine this producing a scenario, where even 50% of those with a variety of learning difficulties could find life a lot easier and less frustrating. And 90% of four-year-olds now entering the education system might never reverse their letters, words and numbers, or develop SpLD.

Let's assume just for a moment that there is nothing wrong with these EPIC students; there is no condition to assess, 'no deficit' to find – only the strengths of being neurodivergent. I believe that progress with many learning difficulties is being limited by trying to answer the wrong question.

We need to change the question away from deficits. We need to stop asking: "Why can't these students learn in the way we are teaching them?" "What is a school doing about testing and remedial action?" and "What is the right age to test my child?" A better question to put our effort into would be something like "How can we best teach a neurodiverse population?" Once you understand mental imagery, the great strengths it brings and the confusion it can generate you can start observing from children just a few months old. We don't want to be continually supporting more students in their confusion when we can be teaching them the skills to work with their strengths and enabling them to excel in their chosen field.

What would this do for our societies worldwide?

When you understand more about students' experiences, the solutions are often frighteningly simple. There are many things you can do to contribute towards these aims and do keep in touch, for any support you need:

- **Pre-birth:** Encourage mothers to have a restful, nurturing pregnancy – even if you have passed this stage, it is never too late to encourage others. Remember what you do may be reflected in your sensitive children.

- **Pre-school:** Talk to your children about their mental images, encourage them to create images when reading a story. Parents can do the "tell a story to mummy/daddy about an elephant." Just picture the elephant and imagine what the elephant is doing and tell your child: "There are no right answers." Then it can be the child's turn. A small child's world is almost all visual. What are the child's interests? What do they love doing? Do they change in a calm environment? Watch their eye movements: Are they anxious or stressed? The more curious you are, the more you will learn before the child is even verbal. Once children are verbal, you can start realising how they use pictures as memory prompts, explaining their experiences, discussing toys, building construction toys and much more. You can get them talking about their pictures, however bizarre they are. So, if they want to picture a blue elephant with pink stripes that is fine. Explore things like the colour of their ears. This will all encourage a brilliant imagination. Getting control is essential. If they get pictures that are scary, use the skills in the book to send them away.

- **Primary School:** Encourage your children and your school to teach mental imagery to every year in school, especially the first year, starting with pictures. Encourage students to keep calm and have control over their mental images, and then they can start adding words and numbers. Encourage parents to improve their skills and understand more about their own children.

- **Secondary school:** First let's change the official office title from the Learning Support Centre to the **Learning Skills Centre**. We need to help struggling students with new skills that match their natural learning strengths. Check how the first year is using or not using their mental images and please ask Empowering Learning for help, and if possible, report your results to them. This data is very valuable to track progress.

- **Secondary School and Adults:** Teach these simple skills. As they go through school, students can develop mental images for all sorts of academic work, sports, art, computer games, storytelling, design, to name just a few. When have you heard someone say a child hasn't got any imagination? Have they ever been encouraged to use it? By the time you have entered the workplace, you may have found visual applications for design, art, writing, architecture, new product development and goal setting. Then you have a family, and the whole cycle starts again – learn the skills for yourself so you can pass them on.

I have no doubt that as soon as this book is published, Empowering Learning will be discovering more information. Through scientific research we expect to put more pieces of the puzzle together about brain development, right-left brain development, primary reflexes, nutrition, pre-, during- and post-birth trauma, the gut, the body's energetic system, delayed chord clamping, multiple brains, the Vegas nerve and much more that contribute to learning differences. All of these are important components to understand EPIC students. I will be returning to my Sherlock Holmes role again, piecing all the clues together and bringing them to the public in a simple and accessible way. But for now I will stop here and you are welcome to keep in contact, through my website www.empoweringlearning.co.uk and especially my blog www.olivehickmott.co.uk where you can find updates on our latest discoveries.

I look forward to having you join us on this adventure.

Additional Assistance

If you need additional help with any part of this book, please contact me, Olive Hikmott, via olive@empoweringlearning.co.uk. This book and associated CDs, downloads, links to programmes/trainings, reference materials, etc. can all be found on www.empoweringlearning.co.uk, which is now part of www.tiahl.org.

Other New Perspectives books for learning include:
Bridges to Success,
Seeing Spells Achieving,
The Jumpstarting Literacy and Numeracy Study Guide.

New Perspectives CDs:
Pass Literacy On
Waldorf – The Dog Who Isn't Word-blind
The Meditations for "Bridges to Success"

As you might expect, there are untold benefits to be derived from working with an experienced coach. I would be delighted to provide any further assistance you might need. We always answer requests for assistance. Also, there is a growing network of international individuals, who can offer local coaching and training. If you are suitably experienced or would like to be trained, please contact me and apply to join the group.

I would also ask readers to provide me with feedback on their experiences so that their interactions can help others.

Please follow me on:
Blog: www.olivehickmott.co.uk, where you will find extensions to this book
Twitter: www.twitter.com/olivehickmott
LinkedIn: www.linkedin.com/in/olivehickmott
Facebook: www.facebook.com/olive.hickmott www.facebook.com/Intassoc

New Perspectives (www.newperspectives.me.uk), has brought together a unique set of books and CDs, for those wishing to explore how they can become the person they want to be. The objective is to offer you tools to start your own personal developmental journey around specific areas on which you're focused, such as:

- *You too can do Health*: Improving general health.
- *Recover your Energy*: Maintaining your energy.
- *Bridges to Success*: Overcoming learning difficulties.
- *Back from the brink …twice*: Coping with Recovery from Intensive Care
- *How to Reduce the Impact of Dementia* - insights for carers.
- Well-being for women CD.
- Recover from physical injury CD.
- Eliminating food intolerances CD.

If you find a particular book or CD of value for an immediate need in your life, you may become curious to understand more about other aspects. We would encourage you to move to other areas that you may feel appropriate. The books have many stories, examples, client experiences, pictures, dialogue and sometime workbook pages to illustrate the point and help you to move forward. They challenge the reader to be open to new perspectives. Personal change is achieved through commitment. Several books employ the healing power of stories that have been passed down through the centuries. As individuals grow within themselves, they find:

- Some of the daily worries of modern living melt away.
- Focus changes to things that are really important.
- A calmer more grounded individual is less affected by negative experience and far more able to cope with challenges.
- Long-term illnesses change and start to shift.
- Energy and fun increase hugely.
- Inner wisdom shines through.

All of the New Perspectives books are designed for "the man/woman in the street"; they work because they just make sense.

Appendix A: Empowering Learning™ Mental Imagery checklist

1. Ask the student to picture something he is very familiar with, i.e. a cat or a dog. How clearly can he see the image?

No image at all	Vague and dim	Moderately clear	Reasonably clear	As vivid as real life

2. What are some other qualities of the image?

Still pictures	Moving all the time	In control of still or moving pictures	The picture is in front of them	The picture is behind them
They are looking down	They are looking up	They look straight-forward	No control i.e., an avalanche of pictures	Stuck in their head

3. When visualising a familiar object, the student gets:

Multiple objects	Multiple TV screens	Objects are fractured	Can recall objects in the fridge	Too close or too far away to see

4. What is the student's creativity and imagination like:

Very creative	Great imagination	Can think out of the box	Drawing/Art is average	Very artistic

5. What is the student's reading like:

Very good	Average	Poor	Hates reading	Doesn't read

6. When the student is reading aloud which of the following statements best describes his experience?

Can read aloud fluently with expression	Not as fluent as reading silently	Stumbles over words when reading aloud	Forgets to breathe at punctuation	Feels very stressed, hates reading aloud

7. When the student is reading which of the following statements best describes what happens to letters and words on the page?

All still with no movement	The word spacing alters, rivers appear "growing" down the page	They are still most of the time unless tired	Some words flash, words move around, letters change places and even fall off the paper	Letters don't stay in straight lines, some move like waves or judder
	Capital letters are easier to read than lower case		Only the current word/line is clear; others go fuzzy.	

8. Which of the following statements best describes the student's ability to recognise nouns/objects words such as cat, lion, table, chair, zebra, window?

Spelling these words is easy	Short familiar words OK. Longer ones difficult	Spelling any words longer than 3 letters is hard	Spelling any words is difficult	Spelling is just guesswork

9. Which of the following statements best describes the student's ability to spell non-object words such as, on, was, sad, close, design, listening, climb?

Spelling these words is easy	Can spell short words I am familiar with, but longer ones are difficult	Spelling any words longer than 3 letters is hard	Spelling any words is difficult	Spelling is just guesswork

10. Which of the following statements best describes the student's ability to spell homophones like their, there, wear, where?

Spelling these words is easy	I don't know which of these words to use	I spell the right one correctly	I sometimes get these correct	They are just guesswork

11. Which of the following statements best describes what happens when the student visualises a letter or a word in his mind's eye?

I can visualise still words	I can visualise still letters	Words fade before I reach the end of the word	Words are too close	The words are too far away to see
I lose bits of the word	Letters don't stay still	When I try to visualise words, all the letters are moving, it is chaos		I can't visualise words

12. Which of the following statements best describes the student's ability to recall what he has read?

I can recall what I read	I can only recall some of what I read	My mind wanders when I am reading, and I forget what I have read	I can't recall anything I read

13. Which of the following statements best describes the student's ability to answer questions about what they have read?

I find it difficult	I find it easy	I find it difficult or slow	I find it really difficult to answer any question	My mind goes blank

14. Which of the following statements best describes what happens when the student is doing mental maths?

I can visualise still numbers	I can do addition, subtraction and multiplication in my mind	The numbers fade before I can complete the calculation	When I try to visualise numbers, they are all moving and its chaos	I can't visualise numbers

Appendix B: Some of the Empowering Learning™ Research

1. Since 2004, thousands of students, across the UK, Ireland, Europe and worldwide have been using these processes following one-to-one sessions with Empowering Learning™practitioners. Many of them have had outstanding success with huge leaps in their spelling, maths and other academic subjects. Many stories of these students are included in this material and in *Bridges to Success*.

2. Empowering Learning™ has worked with the **Dyslexia Research Trust,** which formally assessed nearly 20 students, before and after 2-3 Empowering Learning™ sessions, showing huge improvements across the board. Here is a description of just two cases: An audit from the Dyslexia Research Trust reported on one of Empowering Learning™ student at retest: "He made excellent progress improving single word reading by 2.6 years and single word spelling 2.9 years in just 6 months, with 3 hours of interventions." *"****(7.5 years old) has made dramatic improvements in everything we tested today. It is very unusual for any child to improve their reading and spelling as much as this, in such a short time (6 months). This I believe is all the result of the new teaching method, "picturing" the words and other things in her head. I hope she can continue with her new teacher and keep up the excellent progress".*

3. Three primary schools in Westmeath piloted the project from Oct 2013 – June 2015. The largest of these schools implemented the process in 6-week blocks to assess the impact on various areas. These included; English spelling, Irish spelling, times tables, problem solving in math and reading comprehension. They were delighted with the results and will continue to use this within the school in all classes. More schools and coming on board to run their own trials.

4. The impact of adopting a stress reduction technique and Mental Imagery skills for spelling, on the self-efficacy in learning of adult learners with poor literacy, MA 2013. Sara Haboubi used Empowering Learning™ in her MA research project with adults with poor spelling. This was over a four week period, two hours per week, with great success. A summary of his can be supplied. The literary review is excellent and puts into context many of the diverse views about how people learn to read and spell.

Appendix C: Some of the strengths displayed by Neurodivergent Learners

Creativity, imagination and generation of new ideas

Painters, artists, designers, musicians, film makers, photographers, writers, comedians, etc, – there is reputedly a design house in New York that only employs those with these skills.

Artistic talents are abundant and new ideas appear at lightning speed, sometimes too fast for others to keep up with them!

Inquisitive, creates new designs, even wacky solutions, thinking out of the box.

Problem solving

Thrive on solving problems, puzzles, jigsaw, chess and strategy games. With an interesting problem to solve, they won't be able to drop it until they have found a solution.

Original ideas: Will find creative ways around their learning challenges.

Understands cause and effect, likes to get things right.

Hyperfocus, Drive and Energy

Hyperfocusing enables learners to have single-minded focus on what they consider to be an interesting task or subject.

Concentration on small detail and any changes in detail. Those who focus on minutiae can switch off their peripheral vision, avoiding overload.

Given an interesting project to work on, they are completely absorbed; there is no stopping them!

Resilience

In order to overcome challenges experienced within a conventional learning environment, some will develop a high level of resilience that allows them to focus on their strengths and excel.

Ability to see things from different perspectives, sometimes at the same time.

Can not only imagine what physical objects look like from different perspectives, including cross-sections, they can see, without any difficulty, the other side of an argument, business opportunities that others may not see, etc.

Olive Hickmott has coined the term "Perspectius", meaning an exceptional ability to see different perspectives simultaneously.

Spatial awareness

Ability to turn 2D images into 3D images, e.g. read maps, charts and images easily, when looking at an Ordnance Survey map, which is flat, some people can turn the 2D contour lines into a 3D image of the mountains and hills in their mind's eye.

Memory, collecting, concentrating and connecting facts

Exceptional memory, especially long-term

Noticing patterns in things that others may not see.

A quick thinker, with high speed ability to make connections between different facts.

This enables them to make unusual and unique insights very quickly, without going through a more traditional, slower linear process.

Thinking and learning visually

Thinking in still pictures and videos; this is invaluable for rapid recall and is particularly useful when working in the media.

Extraordinary ability to recall visual memories from movies, video games or actual events.

Drawing in advance of age.

Understands pictures more than words.

Exceptional interpersonal skills.

They display creative verbal communications with rich and interesting advanced vocabulary. May have been developed to make up for their lack of ability with written communication.

Compassion; tremendous powers to connect with other people and in addition an advanced ability to empathise and see different perspectives.

Intuition; they can guide themselves by just knowing, seeing through any façade to the essence of things and people. With intuition goes being highly sensitive, warm-hearted, they see inside people and tend to share their suffering.

Sense of humour; many love to laugh and may have a knack of making others laugh too.

High intelligence.

Many people with dyslexia present with above average intelligence.

Clarity and radical authenticity; a compulsion to be authentic and express their true selves that maybe others find hard to hear. Saying exactly how it is. They see things as they really are, have a strong instinct to question and dismiss information that conflicts with their instincts.

Demonstrates strong opinions / feelings.

Exceptional number skills

Ability to quickly perform complex mental calculations.

May have incredible recall of large amount of data such as dates, timetables and facts and figures around anything that they are interested in.

The bigger picture

Needs to understand the bigger picture and the reasons why, searching out the rationale behind an instruction, needs to verify that it has an authentic purpose or will work to change it.

Asks "big questions," "life's larger questions," challenging questions and questions about how things work.

They believe that everything should be given creative thought, rigid ritualistic systems are considered archaic. Their insights fuel "system busting."

That they have "something special, a unique way of looking at the world, a perspective that others just don't understand, until they meet another – it takes one to recognise one.

Appendix D: References

[1] Art Giser, is the creator of Energetic NLP, www.energeticnlp.com. Energetic NLP is a unique blend of NLP, intuition development and energetic healing and invaluable to my work.

[2] Thought Pattern Management (TPM), created by Robert Fletcher (deceased), Jared Fletcher is the custodian, and European training and development is run by Fiona Sutherland (www.tpmeurope.com). TPM includes Mental Geography and greatly helped my work in this field.

[3] Brian Kinghorn, has several YouTube videos explaining this concept well: Start with Educating in a Neurodiverse World

[4] Functional Medicine is a systems biology–based approach that focuses on identifying and addressing the root cause of disease. Each symptom or differential diagnosis may be one of many contributing to an individual's illness.

[5] Functional Neurology is unpacking the underlying concentrations in childhood developmental disorders, vestibular rehabilitation, and brain injury rehabilitation. Dr. Peter Scire has amassed thousands of hours of continued education in the areas of functional immunology, functional endocrinology and advanced concepts in neurochemistry and nutrition over the past decade. Since 2004, Dr. Scire has collaborated with Dr. Robert Melillo the Founder of Brain Balance Centers and Hemispheric Integration Therapy.

[6] 48XXYY is a genetic disorder, with neurological and mental symptoms, including developmental delays, speech impairment, behavioural issues, social communication disorders, anxiety disorders, depression, learning disability, infertility, mood swings and outbursts and autism spectrum disorders.

[7] Hyperlexia is the obsession with the way a word sounds, with no understanding of the meaning.

[8] Radaker, L. D. (1963), "The Effect of Visual Imagery Upon Spelling Performance," Journal of Educational Research, vol56, 370-2.

[9] From Wikipedia, Educational neuroscience is an emerging scientific field that brings together researchers in cognitive neuroscience, developmental cognitive neuroscience, educational psychology, educational technology, education theory and other related disciplines to explore the interactions between biological processes and education. Researchers in educational neuroscience investigate the neural mechanisms of reading, numerical cognition, attention and their attendant difficulties including dyslexia, dyscalculia and ADHD as they relate to education. The aim of educational neuroscience is to generate basic and applied research that will provide a new transdisciplinary account of learning and teaching, which is capable of informing education.

[10] Dr. Cheri Florance has documented many case studies, including that of her own son, who "had many labels including ADD; autism; mental retardation; learning disabled; multiple-handicapped; deafness and PDD (Pervasive Developmental Disorder). The real problem, as I was to discover, was his over-working visual brain was interfering with the development of his auditory-verbal brain, imitating the symptoms of many of the above disorders. My career as a brain scientist before my son's birth guided me towards this discovery. My subsequent life's work has been devoted to helping other highly visual children and adults to likewise become symptoms free." She has called these highly visual children "Mavericks."

[11] Journal of Educational Research, Vol 56, No7 (March 1963), pp370-372. Neuroscience contributed with the work of Dehaene, Dehaene-Lambert et al in Paris, identifying specific areas in the occipital lobe for recognising faces, building, objects and words, explaining how meaning and pronunciation come first and so much more in *Reading in the Brain.* Stanislas Dehaene's extensive work coined the phrase "The Brain's Letterbox" approach for connections with other areas of the brain.

[12] Drs Sally Shaywitz's and Bennet Shaywitz's, of Yale University, work identified three systems for reading in the brain's left hemisphere. In summary, the work shows a neural pathway from seeing a word on the page to the occipital lobe that takes less than 150msecs to complete for fluent

readers. When seeing a new word, the Broca area, at the front of the brain activates, then the parieto-temporal region for word analysis and on to the occipital temporal region where your "dictionary" is held. The route taken for non-fluent readers stays in the Broca area, trying to understand the letters, phonemes etc, without access to the vital "dictionary" of words seen before that which facilitates word recognition. Shaywitz, Sally E., 1996. Dyslexia. Scientific American. Shaywitz, S. et al Study of Adolescence. Pediatrics 1999, 104:6, pp1351-1359. Shaywitz, Sally, Overcoming Dyslexia, Random House USA Inc; 2005, p79 Dr. Sally E. Shaywitz is a professor of Pediatric Neurology at Yale University.

[13] www.nlpuniversitypress.com, Spelling Strategy P1285-1290, Research P1109. Tom Malloy[13] and F. Loiselle in 1985. More recently various academics have added research: Glezer, Laurie S., Georgetown University Medical Centre Skilled Readers Rely on Their Brain's "Visual Dictionary" to Recognize Words, 2011. The effects of Visual Imagery on Spelling Performance and retention among Elementary Students. Nedra C Sears and Dale M Johnson, University of Tulsa, 2013.

[14] The strategy has been researched by Tom Malloy at the University of Utah and F. Loiselle at the University of Moncton in New Brunswick, Canada 1985. Both research projects showed a significant change in people's ability to spell accurately after learning the NLP Spelling Strategy. These studies support the NLP Spelling Strategy specifically and the NLP notion of Eye-Accessing Cues and Sensory Representation System strategies in general. They are reported in: Dilts, R. and Epstein, T., *Dynamic Learning*, Meta, Capitola, California,1995, and elsewhere in many NLP books. Malloy, Thomas E., Principles of teaching Cognitive Strategies, Dept of Psychology, University of Utah, 2007

[15] www.madebydyslexia.org is a charity championing successful dyslexics, pledging the value of dyslexic thinking #madebydyslexia.

[16] Stephen Wiltshire videos on YouTube. Start with The Human Camera

[17] We are born creative geniuses and the education system dumbs us down, according to NASA scientists. NASA had contacted Dr George Land and Beth Jarman to develop a highly specialized test that would give it the means to

effectively measure the creative potential of NASA's rocket scientists and engineers. The test turned out to be very successful for NASA's purposes, but the scientists were left with a few questions: Where does creativity come from? Are some people born with it or is it learned? Or does it come from our experience? The scientists then gave the test to 1,600 children between the ages of 4 and 5. What they found shocked them. https://ideapod.com/born-creative-geniuses-education-system-dumbs-us-according-nasa-scientists/. Here are the results:

Age 4-5: 98% genius creativity
Age 10: 30% genius creativity
Age 15: 12% genius creativity
Adult: 2% genius creativity

[18] A metaphor: Instagram is a photo and video-sharing social networking service owned by Facebook, Inc.

[19] Youki Terada,published in Edutopia, George Lucas Educational Foundation, *The Science of Drawing and Memory*.

[20] Greta Thunberg , the 16 year-old climate activist demonstrates this perfectly "Asperger's is what makes me different, and being different is a gift. I don't easily fall for lies, I can see through things"

[21] Savants often have one particular ability in a huge amount, such as an exceptional photographic memory.

[22] Indigo children are a new generation of gifted children blessed with supernatural abilities. They are more empathetic beings than previous generations and are drawn to expressing themselves through their creativity. Indigo children are sensitive, curious, independent, open-minded and artistic. Indigo children may ask questions like "Why do we suffer?" "What is the meaning of life?" "Why is there injustice?" "Why was I born?"

[23] www.synesthesiatest.org

[24] *Train the Trainer* programme was a joint venture by the British Dyslexia Association, Dyslexia Action, Manchester Metropolitan University, Helen

Arkel Dyslexia and the Dyspraxia Foundation. Materials available on the BDA web-site.

[25] International Teaching Seminars, NLP Practitioner training, www.itsnlp.com, Ian McDermott

[26] According to M. Zimmerman, 1989 and cited by D William, 2006, P72, The half-second delay: what follows?

Sensory System	Total bandwidth (in bits per spec, BPS)	Conscious bandwidth (in BPS)
Visual	10,000,000	40
Auditory	1,000,000	30
Kinaesthetic	100,000	5
Olfactory	100,000	1
Gustatory	1,000	1

[27] Elevated stress levels raise cortisol levels (stress hormone). Extended periods of raised cortisol levels wither the dendrites in the hippocampus. Information is passed from the Working Memory (WM) to the Long-Term Memory (LTM), and vice versa, via the hippocampus. Therefore, high levels of stress can inhibit memory **and** learning. Reducing stress levels is vital. For some students this is the crucial first step towards improving their learning. Stress affects people's Optimum Learning State that disrupts mental imagery and memory – there is much research. For example: The University of Illinois at Urbana-Champaign, Landscape and Human Health Laboratory. www. http://lhhl.illinois.edu/adhd.htm. The information here is from the original scientific articles:

i. Faber Taylor, A., Kuo, F.E., & Sullivan, W.C. (2001). "Coping with ADD: The surprising connection to green play settings." *Environment and Behavior*, 33(1), 54-77.

ii. Kuo, F.E., & Faber Taylor, A. (2004). "A Potential Natural Treatment for Attention-Deficit/Hyperactivity Disorder: Evidence from National Study." *American Journal of Public Health*, 94(9), 1580-1586.

iii.   Faber Taylor, A. & Kuo, F.E. (2009). "Children with Attention Deficits Concentrate Better after a Walk in the Park." *Journal of Attention Disorders,* 12, 402-409.

[28] Source: Csikszentmihalyi, Mihaly Flow. *Creativity: Psychology of Discovery and Intervention,* New York Harper Perennial, Pronounced Chick-sent-me-hi.

[29] Amanda Spielman, speaking in 2019, at the "Wonder Years" curriculum conference.

[30] The Early Years Foundation Stage was published in 2008, by the Department for Children, Schools and Families. ISBN: 978-1-84775-128-7

[31] The Dame Kelly Holmes Trust, www.damekellyholmestrust.org, gets young lives back on track by using world-class athletes to empower young people facing disadvantages to realise the attitudes they need to fulfil their potential.

[32] Rote learning is learning by constant repetition, like most people learn their time tables.

[33] Professor Adam Zeman, University of Exeter

[34] Wobble cushions are inflated cushions that create instability, encouraging the user to engage their back and core muscles.

[35] Professor Philip Asherson, Kings College London.

[36] David Mitchell's introduction to The Reason I jump by Naoki Higashida

[37] Stimming is an expression used to refer to a number of repetitive movements

[38] The has been much work on the Autonomic Nervous System, what to look out for and the relevance of the Vegus Nerve. Babette Rothschild has published a valuable summary chart, based on the work of Stephen Porges. See also some book references.

[39] Thomas the Tank Engine is a fictional steam locomotive, whose face never changes in The Railway Series of books created by the Reverend Wilbert Awdry.

[40] Grounded for Life , published by Bonnie Landau Weed

[41] There is an article at https://litemind.com/how-to-develop-visualisation-skill/ that has some useful tips.

[42] This slow van featured in Fools and Horses

[43] Simon Baron-Cohen is Professor of Developmental Psychopathology, University of Cambridge and Fellow at Trinity College, Cambridge. He is Director, Autism Research Centre (ARC) in Cambridge.

Referenced further reading

(in alphabetical order)

Allen Sargent: *The Other Mind's Eye*

Arthur and Carly Fleischmann: *Carly's Voice*

Ben Polis: *How I lived with and Triumphed over ADHD*

Brock Eide and Fernette Eide, who published *The Dyslexic Advantage*; one of the first books to identify the advantages of dyslexic skills.

Carol Dweck's invaluable work on *Mindsets* and the need for a growth mindset in all our learning activities.

Cherri Florance, who solved the mystery of her unreachable, unteachable, silent son, now tours the world passing on her valuable experience with what she calls *Maverick Minds and a Boy beyond Reach*.

Claire Wilson, *Grounded*

Clint Ober, Stephen Sinatra, Martin Zucker: *Earthing: The most Important Health Discovery Ever?*

Gail Saltz, whose book *The Power of Different*, links disorders, across the spectrum of mental health, with Genius.

Giulia Enders, *Gut*

Hallowell: *Superparenting for ADD*

Holly Bridges, author of *Reframe your Thinking around Autism. How the polyvagal Theory and Brain Plasticity help us make sense of Autism.*

Howard Glassser, Creator of the Nurtured Heart Approach. His first book *Transforming the Difficult Child* has become a top-selling book on ADHD, providing a heart-centred approach to transforming children without destroying or medicating away their intensity. *Notching Up the Nurtured Heart Approach: The New Inner Wealth Initiative for Educators.* These are the children Howard Glasser refers to as having "Early Onset Greatness."

Ian Robertson: *The Mind's Eye*

Jodi Picoult: *House Rules*

John Heath, his book *When Bright Kids Can't Learn*, highlights the differences between teaching and learning.

John Holt, his book *The Mind's Eye*, led me to many of my early conclusions, "A picture is worth a thousand words, or so they say. However, our education from earliest childhood emphasizes the importance of spoken words, rather than pictures."

Julian G. Elliott, Professor at Durham University, who clearly says that whether a child has a diagnosis of dyslexia or not, the route to success is the same. *The Dyslexia Debate.*

Kabir Jaffe and Ritam Davidson: *Indigo Adults*

Kaufman, *Twice Exceptional*

Ken Robinson, has made so many powerful and persuasive contributions to addressing the impossibility of standardised teaching working for neurodivergent creative students. I love his numerous books and YouTube videos. Books include; *Creative Schools, Finding your Element*

Lee Carroll and Jan Tober: *The Indigo Celebration*

Lucy Wells, *Of the Brain*

Lorrane E Murray, *Calm Kids* and *Connected Kids*

Malcolm Gladwell, *Outliers*

Mark Hyman recently launched *The Broken Brain* series. Mark assembled many experts and much research, primarily on the gut-brain connection for learning differences and also conditions like dementia, depression, MS, etc.

Martha Herbert, whose book *The Autism Revolution*, makes so much sense and shows a new perspective on autism, primarily around the gut.

Math Hadden: *The Curious Incident of the Dog in the Night Time.*

Melvin Kaplan, whose book *Seeing Through New Eyes*, taught me the difference between central and peripheral vision and how it manifests in autism and trauma.

Naoli Higasihida (with introduction from David Mitchell),: *The Reson I Jump*

Norman Doidge, whose book *The Brain that Changes itself*, explains brain plasticity and the science behind it.

Nuala Gardner: *A Friend like Henry*

Oliver Sacks, now sadly deceased, did much research into the mind's eye and published several books, including *The Mind's Eye* and *The Man who Mistook his Wife for an Umbrella*.

Ober, Sinatra, Zucker: *Earthing*

Patrick McKewn talks about the importance of nose-breathing, in *The Oxygen Advantage*.

Radaker L, published *The Effect of Visual Imagery upon Spelling*, 1963, is our oldest reference to mental imagery.

Richard Branson, self-declared dyslexic with ADHD brain, has recently set up a charity called #madebydyslexia, promoting the amazing skills of dyslexics.

Ronald Davis: *The Gift of Dyslexia*

Sally Shaywitz authored *Overcoming Dyslexia*, including MRI scans of the occipital lobe, so important in understanding all aspects of mental imagery.

Stanislas Dehaene and Laurent Cohen identified a region they called the "visual word form area" (VWFA), or "The Brain's Letterbox" that was consistently activated during reading, and Dehaene's book *Reading in the Brain* has extensive explanations, drawn from research.

Stanley Rosenberg, authored Accessing the Healing Power of the Vegus Nerve.

Steve Silberman and his research into the history of autism, Asperger's and neurodiversity, published in *Neurotribes: The legacy of Autism and how to think smarter about people who think differently.*

Temple Grandin, herself autistic and a professor of animal welfare in the USA, uses her exceptional mental images to understand how best to assist cattle. Her books are numerous, and *Thinking in Pictures*, in particular, formulated my early views on mental imagery, where she describes her own experiences with overwhelming mental images. *The Autistic Brain* and *The Way I See it.*

Thomas G West who is an author of three exceptional and well-researched books, including *Seeing What Others Cannot See*, where he explains the revered skills of many highly successful adult dyslexics who are leaders in their field and are fully aware that they think visually. *In the Mind's Eye*, Prometheur books, 1943 and *Thinking like Einstein.*

Printed in June 2019
by Rotomail Italia S.p.A., Vignate (MI) - Italy